Be your own
PERSONAL
TRAINER

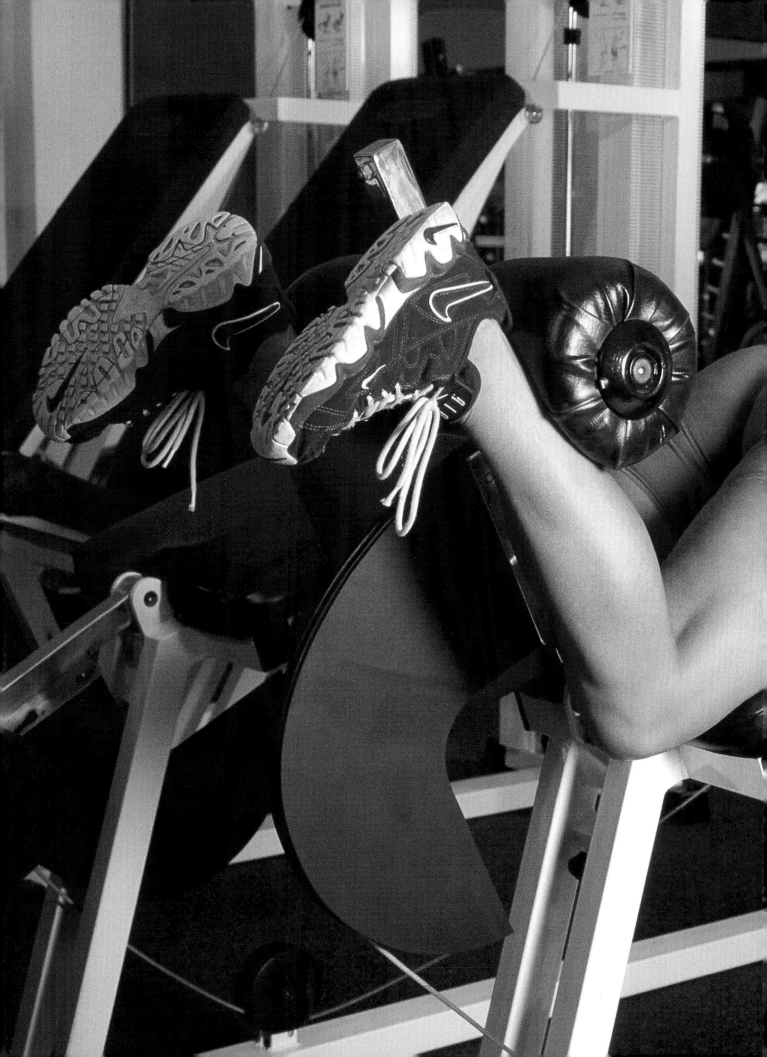

Be your own
PERSONAL
TRAINER

Tanya Wyatt

Published by Silverdale Books
an imprint of Bookmart Ltd in 2005
Bookmart Ltd, Blaby Road, Wigston, Leicester LE18 4SE

Registered Number 2372865

First published in 2004 by New Holland (Publishers) Ltd
London · Cape Town · Sydney · Auckland

www.newhollandpublishers.com

ISBN 1 84509 241 4 (PB)

Publisher: Mariëlle Renssen
Publishing Managers: Claudia Dos Santos, Simon Pooley
Commissioning Editor: Alfred LeMaitre
Studio Manager: Richard MacArthur
Editor: Roxanne Reid
Designer: Lyndall du Toit
Illustrator: Steven Felmore
Picture Researcher: Karla Kik
Production: Myrna Collins
Proofreader: Sandra Cattich
Consultant: Dr Nick Walters, Vice Principal,
                 British College of Medicine

Reproduction by Unifoto, Cape Town, South Africa
Printed and bound in Malaysia by Times Offset
10 9 8 7 6 5 4 3 2 1

DISCLAIMER
Although the author and publishers have made every effort to ensure that the
information contained in this book was accurate at the time of going to press,
they accept no responsbility for any loss, injury or inconvenience sustained by
any person using this book or following the advice given in it.

DEDICATION

To my clients, past and present, who
afford me the experiences that give
life to my knowledge.

Author's note

Welcome to what I hope will be a turning point in your life – an opportunity to take responsibility for your physical self, a time to acknowledge where you are right now and to take a look at your future in terms of your health and fitness.

The aim of this book is to provide you with the tools for lifestyle change: to empower you to move from sedentary being to active doing, and to educate you further about the available choices when you look at what, when and how to exercise. While some people may desire to be physically active in a formal, structured manner – by attending gym sessions regularly, for example – the message I would like to convey is that *all* movement counts, regardless of whether it occurs in your garden, on the beach, in a gym or in your home. In other words, the traditional structure of disciplined training can take a back seat; in its place you can have more fun with physical activity, learn to empower and trust yourself with regard to healthy lifestyle choices and start listening to your body in relation to the most suited type of activity for your genetic makeup.

My hope is that after you have read this book you will be able to develop your own unique and individualized physical activity programme – one that will fully suit your lifestyle, for you can never hope to change successfully unless the change is sustainable and, above all, enjoyable.

For those of you ready to make the change – good luck with the process and remember to honour and acknowledge yourself for such a positive decision. For those of you simply considering the possibility of change, and using this book to inform yourselves about the process you might only undertake sometime in the future – I hope to encourage you to take the first of many small steps that will lead to an active life filled with vigour. Finally, to those who are already converted and want only to further their knowledge by reading such a book – I salute you, not only for the positive choices you made in becoming active, but for your desire to remain informed about what is arguably the most important aspect of optimal health.

Enjoy.

Acknowledgements

Many thanks to Bruce McLoughlin for offering his vast knowledge so willingly; also to Drummond Murphy (Woolworths), Tanya de Kock (Falke) and Belinda Reid (Triumph) for their input. Gratitude, respect and a great deal of love to Sally Lee and Mark Vella, dear friends and colleagues, for their unending inspiration, support and input.

To my models – Stuart, Paul, Glennis, Mike and Nikki – you are all gorgeous and add something special to my book. Many thanks, too, to Virgin Active, particularly Linda Holmes and Steve Murray, for organizing the venue for our shoot, and to Paul Underwood for doing the same in his studio.

To Alfred LeMaitre, Roxanne Reid, Lyndall du Toit and Danie Nel, and everyone I have been involved with at New Holland Publishing, thank you for your hard work and support, and for providing me with such a fantastic experience.

Huge thanks and love to Stu for his utter and complete faith in my abilities, as well as for his incredible support. And last, but not least, thanks to my beautiful, supportive family for engendering in me the self-assurance and confidence to know that I can do anything I put my mind to!

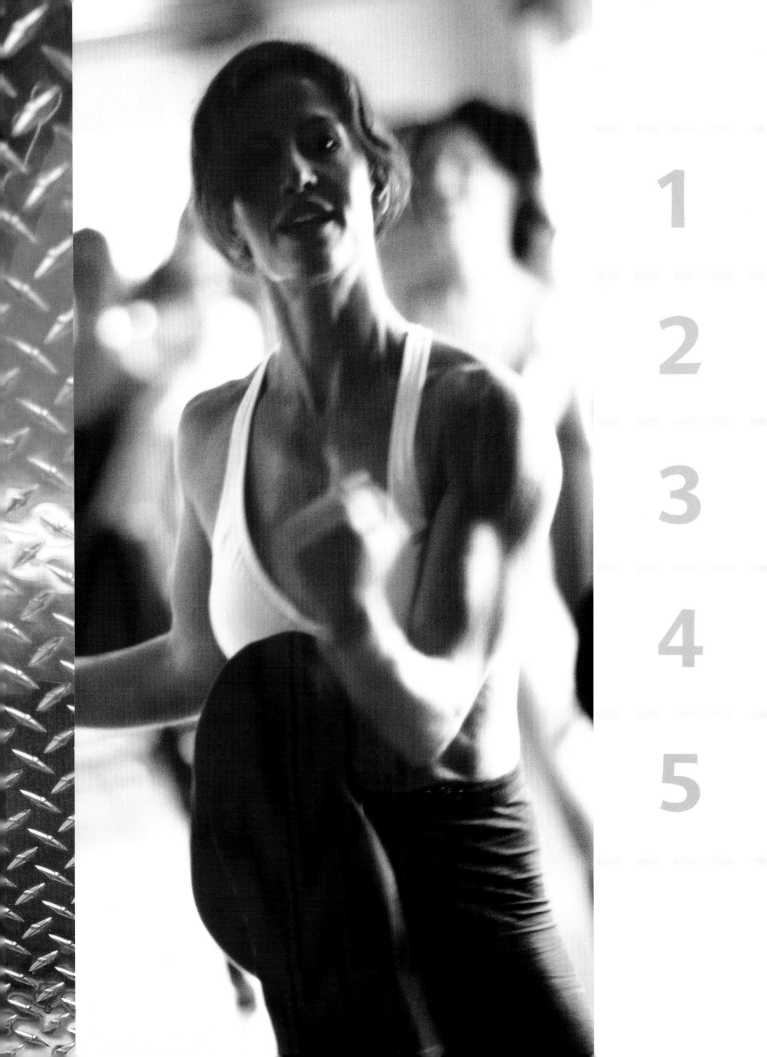

1
2
3
4
5

CONTENTS

Exploring health and habits

Health is defined by the World Health Organization as 'physical, mental, social, spiritual and emotional wellbeing; not just the absence of disease'. In other words, you cannot assume that you are healthy simply because you show no signs and symptoms of illness or disease. Addressing all facets of your being in a holistic manner will bring you closer to the point of true *wellness*.

In the same way, being physically fit does not necessarily mean that you are healthy. For instance, if you are capable of running a marathon but you smoke and eat poorly, you would not be considered as healthy as someone who can only run two kilometres but who has a lifestyle that supports the concept of true health.

Improving your health and fitness will, among other things, reduce your risk of developing diseases that are linked to inactivity. Although this requires an investment of time and energy, the benefits are substantial from both a health and financial point of view

– think how much you could save on medical expenses. You can achieve this improvement in your health by modifying your lifestyle and behaviour, and by adjusting your mindset and attitude towards physical activity.

The diagram below, taken from the Exercise Teachers Academy's Manual for Fitness Professionals, represents your health continuum. You will notice that the area to the left of centre deals with illness, while the area on the right deals with optimal health. Although it certainly makes sense to keep yourself to the right of centre, many people seem unable to achieve this either through a lack of knowledge or lack of motivation. Health enhancement is the first of many steps towards personal wellness and can be initiated anywhere along this continuum.

Health Continuum

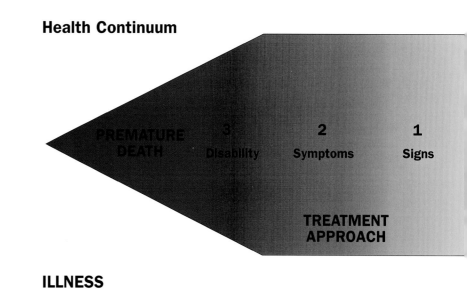

PREMATURE DEATH
3 Disability
2 Symptoms
1 Signs

TREATMENT APPROACH

ILLNESS

Although the idea of being able to take responsibility for your own health can be very empowering, it can also be daunting, so it is imperative that you begin the process gradually – taking little steps, one at a time.

Physical activity is defined as movement performed by the body involving the skeletal muscles, and resulting in an increase in energy output. This book will focus on health-related physical activity and fitness, as opposed to perfomance-related fitness.

Optimal physical fitness, as described by the American Council on Exercise, is 'the condition resulting from a lifestyle that leads to the development of an optimal level of cardiovascular endurance, muscular strength and flexibility, as well as the achievement of ideal body weight'. In other words, being fit – from the point of view of health – should allow you to pursue daily activities with vigour and enthusiasm, and with enough energy left over for leisure activities, hobbies, sports, and so on.

Cardiovascular endurance (also called cardiorespiratory endurance, or aerobic fitness) is the ability of your heart, lungs and blood vessels to deliver the appropriate amount of oxygen to your working muscles.

Muscular strength is the maximum amount of force a muscle or group of muscles can produce in a single contraction, while *muscular endurance* is the number of repeated contractions a muscle or group of muscles can produce against a load without becoming tired. It could also describe the amount of time a contraction can be held without fatiguing. Both are achieved by means of resistance training, which is when muscles contract against a load or resistance.

Flexibility refers to the range of motion around your joints.

What are the benefits?

Some of the benefits of physical activity and fitness have already been noted, and many more that relate specifically to cardiovascular fitness, resistance and flexibility training are listed in Chapter Three. In a nutshell, however, physical activity helps to:
• reduce the effects of ageing;
• improve circulation;
• control body weight more effectively;
• improve body awareness;
• decrease the risk of lifestyle diseases;
• improve immune system function.

Apart from these physiological benefits, however, there are also psychological benefits. Knowing about these may motivate you to make the move towards a more active lifestyle. Physical activity also helps to:
• reduce anxiety, depression and stress;
• increase self-esteem and confidence;
• make you feel more mentally alert, effective and productive in your job and life in general.

What about nutrition?

The role of nutrition should not be underestimated. While it is essential for health that you exercise frequently, it is imperative that you acknowledge the impact, whether positive or negative, that your chosen manner of eating will have on your health. Many people seem uncomfortable with the responsibility that this places on them, choosing instead to try various potions, lotions, pills and

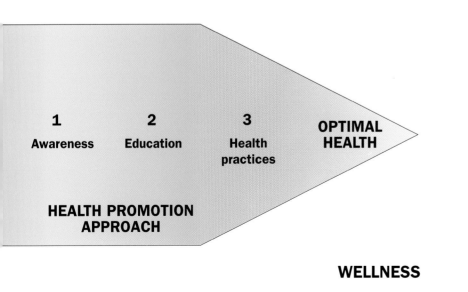

1
Awareness

2
Education

3
Health practices

OPTIMAL HEALTH

HEALTH PROMOTION APPROACH

WELLNESS

treatments in an attempt to bypass this responsibility.

Fad diets promising quick fixes do not support a healthy lifestyle; indeed, they move you further and further away from true health and self-empowerment. In order to achieve optimal health through nutrition, hard work is required but remember that the benefits you will reap in fact far outweigh the effort.

Although the focus of this book is on physical activity rather than nutrition, the following guidelines are important.

- Keep as close to nature as possible – choose whole foods over processed ones.
- Eat a variety of foods.
- Drink at least six to eight glasses of water daily, preferably filtered or bottled if water quality is an issue in your country. Drink more if you are active.
- Avoid saturated fats and include more omega-3 and omega-6 fats in your diet (for example, seeds and their cold-pressed oils; avocados; nuts; deep-water fish and their oils).
- Avoid sugar, salt and alcohol as much as possible.
- Eat as many raw foods as possible. If cooking is necessary, use steaming, grilling, baking or steam-frying.
- Choose foods lower on the glycaemix index (*see* table, right), since these tend not to spike blood sugar levels. Increases in blood sugar lead to increased insulin production, which may, in turn, lead to increased body fat storage.

GLYCAEMIC INDEX

Scale: 0 — 25 — 50 — 75 — 100

PULSES
- Baked beans
- Butter beans
- Chick peas
- Blackeye beans
- Haricot beans
- Kidney beans
- Lentils
- Soya beans

DAIRY PRODUCTS
- Ice cream
- Yoghurt
- Whole milk
- Skimmed milk

VEGETABLES
- Cooked parsnips
- Cooked carrots
- Instant potato
- New potatoes
- Cooked beetroot
- Peas

SUGARS
- Glucose
- Maltose
- Lucozade
- Honey
- Mars Bar
- Sucrose (sugar)
- Fructose

FRUIT
- Raisins
- Bananas
- Orange juice
- Oranges
- Apples

Foods with the greatest effect on blood sugar have the highest score. Try to choose foods with a GI of less than 50, which release sugars into the bloodstream more slowly.

GLYCAEMIC INDEX (cont)

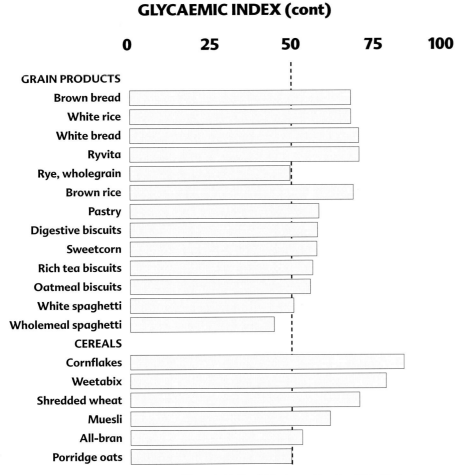

GRAIN PRODUCTS
- Brown bread
- White rice
- White bread
- Ryvita
- Rye, wholegrain
- Brown rice
- Pastry
- Digestive biscuits
- Sweetcorn
- Rich tea biscuits
- Oatmeal biscuits
- White spaghetti
- Wholemeal spaghetti

CEREALS
- Cornflakes
- Weetabix
- Shredded wheat
- Muesli
- All-bran
- Porridge oats

Reproduced with kind permission of Patrick Holford (*Optimum Nutrition Bible*, Piatkus)

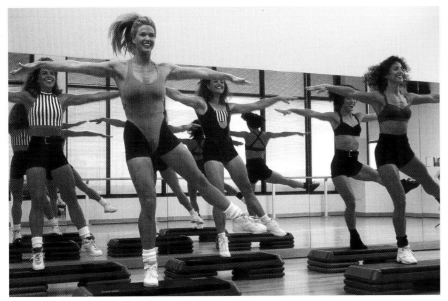

High-intensity aerobics helps to burn calories and raise your metabolism.

- Avoid foods that contain growth hormones, steroids, colourants, flavourants, preservatives and sweeteners.
- Do not overeat; rather eat smaller meals more frequently. A meal could consist of something as simple as fruit and a handful of nuts.
- Do not try to be perfect. Note that these guidelines advise you to 'avoid', not 'cut out altogether'. It would be no fun at all – nor would it be sustainable over time – if you were never to experience deliciously decadent desserts again. Do splash out, but support these not-so-healthy choices by keeping a good 75–80 per cent of your diet 'clean'.

What is the skinny on fat burning?

One of the first questions asked by new exercisers who are looking to get lean is: 'What type of activity should I do to burn the most fat?' The answer is: 'All of them.' The truth is that there are many different ways in which you can look at tackling this issue.

1. **High-intensity aerobic activity** burns large amounts of energy (calories), using muscle glycogen as its main fuel source. Most importantly, your metabolism will be raised significantly both during the activity and for a limited period afterward. This type of workout equates to a short, hard exercise session, such as an indoor cycling class, a kickboxing workout, or fast jogging. Suggested time is 30–60 minutes a session.

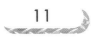

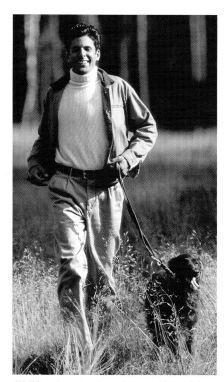

Walking is a low-intensity aerobic activity.

Drawback: the amount of energy and motivation required to complete the session
Benefit: it is over quickly and you have moved one step closer to improving your fitness level

2. **Low-intensity aerobic activity** will use fat as its predominant source of fuel and so will burn fat directly, to a large extent bypassing muscle glycogen. This equates to a long, easy exercise session, for instance, at least 45 minutes of walking, slow cycling on even ground, or easy swimming. Suggested time is 60 minutes or more.
Drawback: time consuming
Benefit: no huge amount of energy required for you to complete the session

3. **Resistance training** results in increased lean muscle mass, thus changing both your body composition and your metabolism (*see* page 36).
Drawback: consistency and commitment, in order to achieve results
Benefit: more lean muscle mass, which burns more energy at rest

So, in general, high- and low-intensity aerobic activities are short-term approaches to fat burning, while resistance training provides you with a long-term approach. It figures, then, that your best bet would be to engage in both cardiovascular (aerobic) and resistance training, combined with a healthy eating plan if fat loss is a personal goal. Just be sure you do not try to lose weight too quickly by being extreme with your programme. A loss of just 0.5kg (1 lb) per week is a sure way

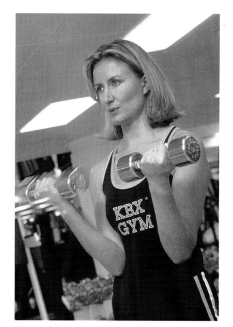

Use weights to increase lean muscle mass.

to keep it off; anything faster may simply be water loss or, even worse, loss of muscle tissue. Since muscle weighs more than fat, you may pick up weight as you begin an exercise programme, particularly one that includes resistance training. Do not be discouraged, as you could be shedding excess body fat at the same time. Try not to focus on your weight but judge by how your clothes feel on you, and how you feel about yourself in general. Be aware, too, that you may start to notice an increase in muscle size before you notice a decrease in body fat, and this may make your clothes feel tight. Be patient – give yourself a couple of months before you start to assume the worst. If you persevere, you will start to see some impressive changes.

Good habits, bad habits

Stress is something we all know about and have no doubt experienced at some point in our lives. Although the term covers a wide range of both positive events (for example, exercise can be perceived as a stress by the body) and negative events (for example, missing a deadline), for the purposes of this section, a stressor is defined as something that is negatively perceived by the person who is experiencing it.

Stressors play a significant role with regard to habits. A habit is a repetitive pattern of behaviour that is unconscious or at least has a low level of consciousness, and is triggered by certain events or circumstances that may involve a stressor. Habits can either be *health enhancing* – for example, exercising when feeling angry, or meditating when feeling anxious – or *health damaging* – for example, smoking when you are pressured for time, drinking alcohol or eating for comfort when you are feeling depressed.

It would be helpful to know yourself well enough to understand your habits and what triggers them. In the examples of negative habits given above, the triggers were stress and depression. Being conscious of the fact that these two triggers result in smoking, drinking alcohol or comfort eating could help you make a different behavioural decision the next time round. An alternative would be to go for a brisk walk around the block to help release some stress, or to talk to a good friend or a counsellor when you feel depressed.

It is vital that you find feasible and realistic ways of changing your behaviour so that these changes do not have a negative impact on your life. For example, do not choose to go for a run or walk when you are feeling stressed if you dislike both activities; rather look for an activity you will enjoy, so that the new association between stress and physical activity is a positive one.

Keep a diary for a couple of weeks, noting both events that evoke a response in you, as well as your resultant behaviour. You may start to notice a pattern, and seeing this pattern on paper should help you to understand whether your habits support a healthy lifestyle or are detrimental

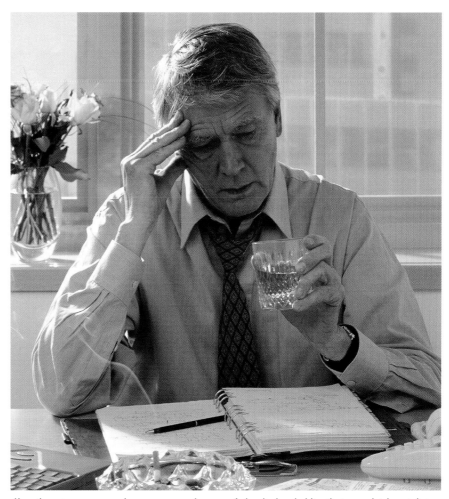

Negative stressors may increase your chances of developing habits that are detrimental to your health – such as smoking and drinking too much alcohol.

to your health. From here, you could develop a plan of action with specific goals and relevant time frames for changing any negative habits (*see* page 52). Remember to be gentle with yourself when trying to change habits. As Mark Twain remarked: 'A habit is a habit and not to be flung out of the window by any man, but coaxed downstairs a step at a time.'

Examples of positive behaviour choices you can make in response to stressful situations include physical activity, meditation, expression of feelings, sleeping, going for a massage, attending a relaxation class or just doing something fun, which is something we often forget about. While some of these may not be appropriate at the time you are experiencing the stress, others may be. The trick is to find the most effective possible way of dealing with a stressor at the time, or shortly after it occurs, as stress has an accumulative impact on your health.

What is your body type?

There are three basic body shapes: mesomorph, ectomorph and endomorph. In between these three lie 'blends' of their characteristics – endo-meso or meso-endo, meso-ecto or ecto-meso.

A good way to determine which of the three body types you are is to clasp your thumb and middle finger of one hand around the wrist of your other arm. If your finger overlaps your thumb, it is likely that you are an ectomorph. Should your fingers touch, chances are you are a mesomorph. If they do not touch at all, you are probably an endomorph.

Look at the diagram below and decide where you think your body shape currently lies. Then note the characteristics listed below in order to get a better idea of your body type traits. If you feel you want to change your shape, look at your current body type on this scale and then identify what you think your (realistic) ideal is. As long as they are not on opposite ends of the scale, the body shape between these two is perhaps an achievable goal.

Mesomorph: You are generally muscular, with shoulders broader than your waist. Your abdomen tends to be firm and your hips

TYPICAL MALE AND FEMALE BODY SHAPES OF ENDOMORPHS, MESOMORPHS AND ECTOMORPHS

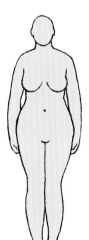
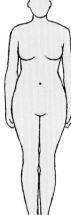
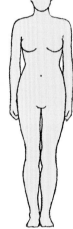
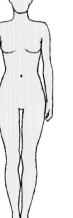
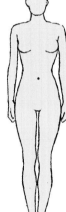
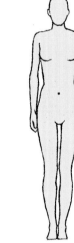
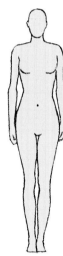

Endomorph	Endo-meso	Meso-endo	Mesomorph	Meso-ecto	Ecto-meso	Ectomorph

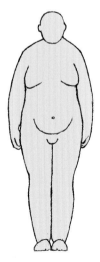
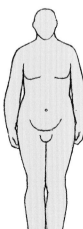
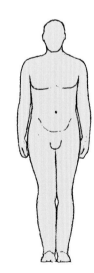
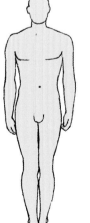
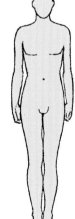
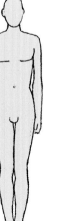
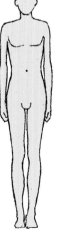

narrow. Your lower extremities are fairly toned and defined. Although you may have a tendency to store as much fat as you have muscle, losing excess body fat is not as difficult as it is for other types, due to a high ratio of muscle mass and thus a high metabolism. You are usually a natural when it comes to learning new sports or physical activities requiring athletic skill.

You would do well to engage in a general exercise programme that offers a variety of intensities and activities, incorporating cardio-vascular, resistance and flexibility training. As far as sports go, you would tend towards those that involve power, strength and short energy bursts, such as rugby, boxing, gymnastics, sprinting and martial arts.

Ectomorph: You are generally quite slim, with long extremities and a narrow pelvis. You tend to have less fat and muscle than the other two body types and, due to a naturally high metabolic rate, struggle to put on weight and/or muscle mass. This does not mean, however, that you should not exercise or that you will by definition have a healthy body composition. You should still exercise to ensure optimal health. Although naturally gravitating towards endurance activities, you would benefit from including some resistance training for muscle strength. Sports you may enjoy include volleyball, basketball, ballet, long-distance running and diving.

Endomorph: You generally store a high amount of body fat due to a naturally slower metabolism. Fat

tends to be stored around either your waist or buttocks and thighs. With a strong body from carrying extra weight, you do well with strength activities and may thus enjoy sports that use your size beneficially, such as wrestling, weight lifting, rugby or suspended water sports (your flotation is good, due to a higher percent-age of more buoyant body fat).

You would do well on a cardiovascular programme that initially encourages a lower intensity and longer duration, coupled with a resistance training pro-gramme for muscle endurance to reduce excess body fat.

What is your main muscle fibre type?

Muscles consist of individual muscle fibres, which contract either slowly or quickly, making them what we call *slow twitch* (ST) or *fast twitch* (FT) fibres respectively. Everyone has both types of muscle fibres, but genetics gener-ally determine the ratio.

People with a high number of FT fibres excel in activities requiring short, sharp bursts of energy, such as shotput or sprinting, while those with ST fibres do well in activities requiring endurance, such as marathon running or long-distance cycling. These fibre types use different energy systems within the body. Simply put, ST fibres use mainly an oxygen-dependent sys-tem, while FT fibres use mainly an oxygen-independent system. Some activities require the use of a com-

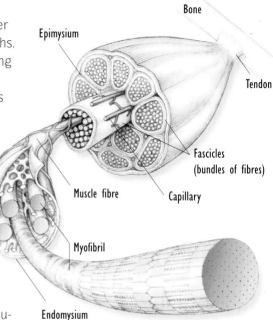

Knowing what your predominant muscle fibre type is will help you to understand what activities are best suited for you.

bination of both types of energy system and so both types of fibres will, to some degree, be activated and trained.

To determine which fibre type is predominant in your body, you could go the truly scientific route and have a muscle biopsy per-formed. During this procedure, medical staff will extract a small sample of muscle so that its make-up can be studied.

Alternatively, if you would prefer to avoid pain at all costs, you will probably find that you naturally gravitate towards the activities that are most com-fortable or enjoyable to you. Although this is not terribly scientific, it may in a sense indicate the predominance of the fibre types in your body.

Assessing **yourself**

This chapter describes various assessments relating to different aspects of physical activity. Some assess your willingness to change your current lifestyle to one that includes more physical activity; others assess you in a more hands-on, physical manner. Everyone should complete the pre-participation health screening assessment. Try to complete the rest of the assessments as well, or at least those you feel are relevant to you and your health and fitness goals.

These assessments will provide you with a starting point; retesting yourself against these results in future can be a great motivator for programme continuance. The latter part of this chapter will help you score against the questions asked opposite, and give you a better understanding of where you and your body are right now.

Since many of the muscles' scientific names are used in the scoring section (these terms being more concise than descriptions in layman's terms), check them against the muscle descriptors in Chapter Four (*see* pages 56–59) for a better understanding of where they all are in your body.

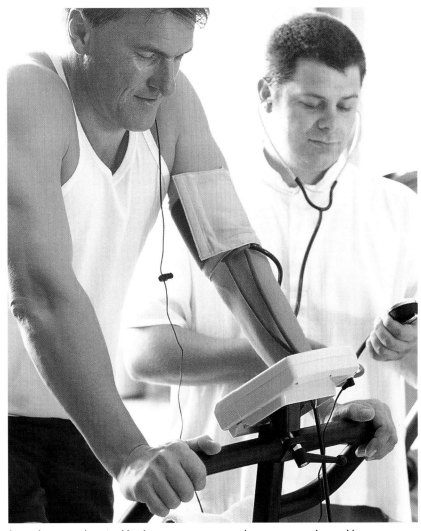

A monitor records your blood pressure as you work out on a cycle machine.

Assessing:

Pre-participation health screening

(Scoring on pages 24—29)

1. Are you male and above the age of 45? Y N

2. Are you female and above the age of 55? Y N

3. Does your family have a history of heart attacks or sudden death before the age of 55 in your father or any other first-degree male relative (i.e. brother or son); or before 65 in your mother or any other first-degree female relative (i.e. sister or daughter)? Y N

4. Do you currently smoke, or have you quit within the last six months? Y N

5. Is your blood pressure over 140/90mm Hg (taken at least twice, on separate occasions) or are you on antihypertensive (high blood-pressure reducing) medication? Y N

6. Is your total serum cholesterol more than 200mg/dL (5.2mmol/L), or is your high-density lipoprotein (HDL) less than 35mg/dL (0.9mmol/L)? Y N

7. Have you been diagnosed with insulin-dependent diabetes mellitus? Y N

8. Are you currently physically inactive? Y N

9. Have you been advised not to exercise by a health-care professional (such as a physician, naturopath, etc.)? Y N

10. Do you have a condition or injury that may be aggravated by physical activity? Y N

11. Are you pregnant or have you given birth in the last three months? Y N

12. Do you know of any other reason why you should not do physical activity? Y N

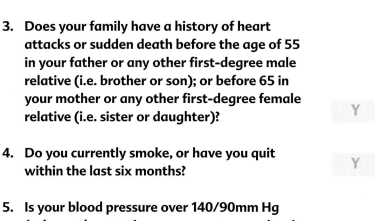

Use weight and height measurements to calculate BMI.

Lifestyle assessment

Assessing your readiness to change is arguably one of the most important aspects of this chapter. You can develop the most wonderfully balanced and effective physical activity programme but without commitment to it and passion for it, it is not worth the paper on which it is written. Be as truthful as you can when answering these questions — if you are truly not ready for a lifestyle change, it would be far more beneficial to acknowledge that fact and perhaps try to discover what is holding you back.

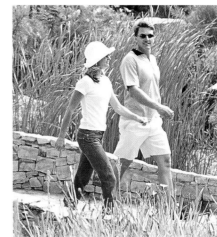

Answer either A or B, depending on whether your goal is to get fit (A — this automatically includes health benefits), or simply to promote your health (B). Then complete the rest of the section (C and D).

A. Health and fitness benefits (p24)

1. I have time in my day to dedicate 30 to 60 minutes to exercising at one time.   AGREE   DISAGREE

2. I have time in my week to dedicate between three and seven days to exercising for 30 to 60 minutes at one time.   AGREE   DISAGREE

3. I am prepared to work at a moderate to high intensity during my exercise sessions.   AGREE   DISAGREE

B. Health benefits (p24)

1. I have time in my day to dedicate 30 minutes or more to physical activity, even if I have to complete two 15-minute or three 10-minute sessions at a time.   AGREE   DISAGREE

2. I have time in my week to include daily physical activity at least five times, even if that daily activity happens in shorter sessions, as described above.   AGREE   DISAGREE

3. I am able to get up 10 to 15 minutes earlier in the morning in order to be physically active for that period.   AGREE   DISAGREE

4. I am able to take 10 to 15 minutes during lunchtime in order to be physically active for that period.   AGREE   DISAGREE

5. I am able to put aside 10 to 15 minutes in the evening in order to be physically active for that period.   AGREE   DISAGREE

C. Support (p24)

1. I have a friend, spouse, partner to offer me emotional support while I implement lifestyle changes to become more physically active.   AGREE   DISAGREE

2. I have a friend, spouse, partner or relative who can offer me support in the form of a training partner, at all or some of my training sessions.

AGREE   DISAGREE

3. I know of a group exercise class (for example, a group of runners, cyclists or swimmers, or an aerobics class) I can join if I feel the need to be motivated.

AGREE   DISAGREE

4. I have a role model in mind to help me adhere to and remain motivated about my programme.

AGREE   DISAGREE

D. Mindset (pp24–25)

1. I enjoy physical activity.

AGREE   DISAGREE

2. I have always been physically active in some way, even if intermittently through my life.

AGREE   DISAGREE

3. I choose to be physically active because it is my desire to be.

AGREE   DISAGREE

4. Being physically active makes me feel more mentally alert and capable.

AGREE   DISAGREE

5. Being physically active helps to make me feel good about my physical self.

AGREE   DISAGREE

6. Being physically active makes me feel as though I have some control over my health.

AGREE   DISAGREE

7. I choose to become physically active because I know I should.

AGREE   DISAGREE

8. I choose to become physically active because someone (physician, spouse, partner or other) has said that I must.

AGREE   DISAGREE

9. I do not believe that being physically active will make that much difference to my state of mind.

AGREE   DISAGREE

10. I do not feel it is that important to have control over my own health, since I believe that to be the role of my physician.

AGREE   DISAGREE

11. I have never experienced a sense of improvement in my physical being through exercise.

AGREE   DISAGREE

12. My overall health and wellbeing is not really all that important to me right now.

AGREE   DISAGREE

Muscle balance (p25)

There are generally three types of postures presented by people (*see* illustrations, below). Since the position of the pelvis often dictates what happens further up or down the body in terms of muscle balance or imbalance, it is the focal point of any postural assessment. This section will help you determine some of your own postural balances and imbalances. While it is not an in-depth assessment – which would require a trained practitioner to apply a series of muscle strength and flexibility tests on you – it should allow you to pick up fairly obvious issues relating to your posture. Use the information contained in both Chapter Three (Planning your Programme) and Chapter Four (The Exercise Menu) to develop your own unique rebalancing programme.

Stand sideways in front of a mirror in what feels like a naturally relaxed position — that is, do not try to stand with perfect posture. Place two fingers of the hand furthest from the mirror onto your pubic bone, making sure you can actually feel the bone. Place two fingers of your other hand onto the top of the hipbone of the leg closest to the mirror. Check to see if the fingers on your hipbone are further in front of the fingers on your pubic bone (anterior pelvic tilt), further behind them (posterior pelvic tilt) or in line with each other (neutral pelvis). Note your position in the diagrams below. These demonstrate extreme positions to show clearly the different pelvic tilts; yours may be far more subtle.

MUSCLE BALANCE QUIZ

Circle the most relevant answer (noted in *italics*):

1

My pelvis is in the *neutral / anterior / posterior* position and *is / is not* lop-sided to the *left / right*.

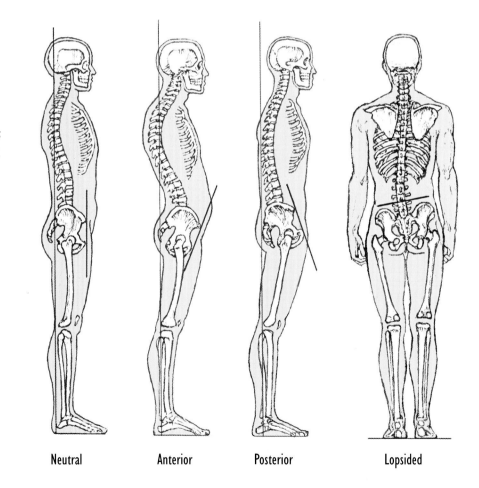

Neutral   Anterior   Posterior   Lopsided

Now face the mirror (again, in a naturally relaxed position) and mark off your observations below:

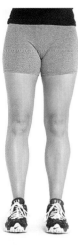 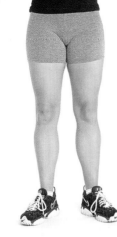 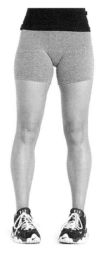

My legs and feet are *facing forward / externally* (outwardly) *rotated / internally* (inwardly) rotated.

Legs/feet facing forward   Legs/feet externally rotated   Legs/feet internally rotated

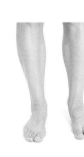 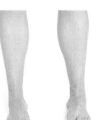

The ankle of my *right / left* foot falls *inward / outward*.

Right foot falls inward   Ankles fall outward

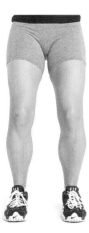 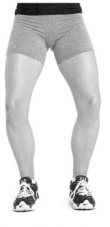

When I bend my knees to 45 degrees, my knees roll *inward / outward* (the point of reference being the middle toes).

Straight bent knees   Knees roll inward   Knees roll outward

21

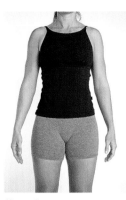
Neutral arms

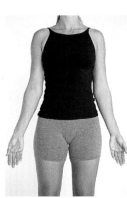
Arms externally rotated

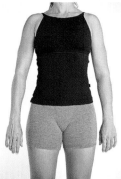
Arms internally rotated

5

My arms and hands are in a *neutral position* (palms facing legs / *externally rotated* / *internally rotated* (*see* left).

Now stand sideways again and look at yourself in the mirror, being careful not to change your posture as you turn your head:

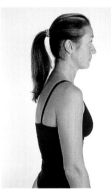
Shoulders droop forward

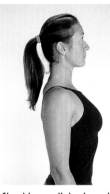
Shoulders roll backward

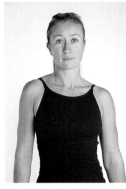
Lop-sided shoulders

6

My shoulders are *drooping forward* / *rolling backward* / *lopsided to the left* / *right* (*see* left).

7

My upper back is *rounded* / *straight* (*see* far left and middle).

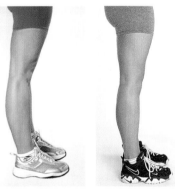
Knees behind hips   **In line with hips**

8

My knees fall *behind* / *in line with* my hips (*see* right).

9

My shoulder blades *stick out of* / *are flat against* my back.

10

My ears fall *in front of* / *in line with* my neck.

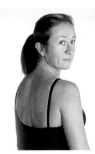
Flat shoulder blades

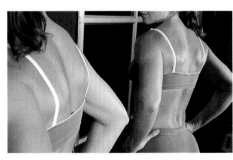
Shoulder blades stick out

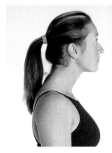
Ears in front of neck

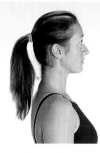
Ears in line with neck

Exercise preference (p27)

	AGREE	DISAGREE
1. I enjoy activities that make me feel out of breath through continuous, repetitive action for more than 10 minutes .	AGREE	DISAGREE
2. I enjoy activities that make me sweat but do not involve continuous, repetitive action over a longer duration.	AGREE	DISAGREE
3. I enjoy activities that make my body feel it is being stretched.	AGREE	DISAGREE
4. I enjoy activities that involve choreography.	AGREE	DISAGREE
5. I enjoy activities performed to the beat of music.	AGREE	DISAGREE
6. I enjoy activities that require a high degree of skill.	AGREE	DISAGREE
7. I enjoy solo activities.	AGREE	DISAGREE
8. I enjoy group activities.	AGREE	DISAGREE
9. I enjoy repetitive activities.	AGREE	DISAGREE
10. I enjoy activities that change mode frequently.	AGREE	DISAGREE
11. I enjoy activities that require a stop / start action.	AGREE	DISAGREE

Cardiovascular fitness (p28)

This section offers you the chance to find out just how strong or weak your heart is. The test used here comes from the Cooper Institute and requires you to time yourself as you walk or run a distance of 2.5km (1.5 miles) on flat ground. Bear in mind that issues such as weather conditions, energy levels and motivation can all impact significantly on the outcome of this test, so try to be as consistent as possible when using it.

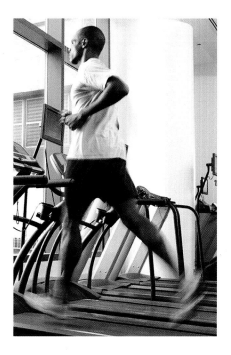

Right: Walking is a good low-impact, inexpensive way to become fitter.

Body composition (p29)

Body mass index (BMI) is used to assess your weight relative to your height. It is calculated by dividing your body weight in kilograms by your height in metres squared. (To convert pounds into kilograms, divide by 2.205; to convert inches into metres multiply by 0.0254.) For example, if your weight is 80kg and your height is 1.8m, your height squared is 3.2m. Divide 80kg by 3.2m and your BMI is 25.

Where body fat is stored reveals a great deal about whether or not a person is currently obese, or at risk of obesity, and the diseases associated with it. People with

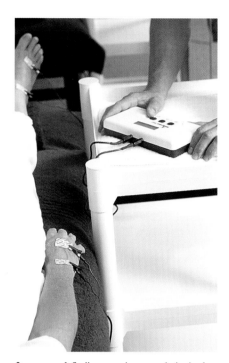

One way of finding out how much body fat you have is to have it tested electronically.

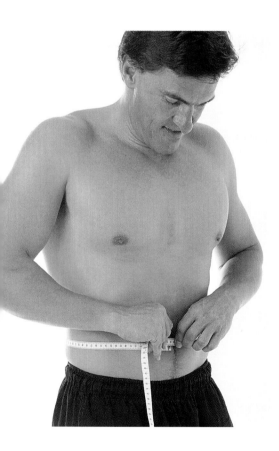

Left: Your waist measurement can indicate your risk of obesity and associated diseases.

more fat stored around their trunks, particularly abdominal fat, are more at risk of developing diseases, such as high blood pressure, diabetes, coronary heart disease and premature death, than others who may carry the same amount of fat, but store more of it in their arms or legs.

A *waist circumference* measurement can thus be used to determine abdominal obesity. For accuracy's sake, measure a point halfway between the bottom of your rib cage and the top of your hipbone – this will indicate the point around which you should take your measurement, in centimetres or inches.

Scoring:
Pre-participation health screening (p17)

These questions cover factors *that can be changed*, such as smoking, inactivity, high blood pressure, and so on, as well as those that *cannot be changed*, such as age, gender and hereditary health problems. If you answered yes to to or more of these questions, it is important that you seek clearance by your health-care professional before beginning a physical activity programme. Equally, if you are unsure of your own blood pressure or cholesterol values, or if you have not had a medical checkup in the past year, do go and visit your health-care professional anyway, so that he or she can test these for you.

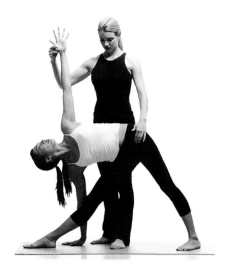

Lifestyle assessment (pp18-19)
A. Health and fitness benefits

If you answered 'agree' to all three questions, you show commitment to initiating or maintaining a lifestyle that encourages the promotion of health and fitness, through physical activity.

B. Health benefits

If you answered 'agree' to at least three questions, you are on the road to improving your health through the incorporation of physical activity.

C. Support

If you answered 'agree' to at least two of the questions, you can feel fairly confident about the likelihood of your programme's success, since motivation and support are imperative for adherence.

D. Mindset

Questions 1–6: Answering even one 'agree' here indicates that you have the motivation to be physically active. Well done.

Questions 7–10: Answering even one 'agree' here indicates that it may be very difficult for you to remain motivated to adhere to your programme. Reassess both your goals and your motivation, since without personal buy-in to your physical activity programme it is highly unlikely that you will feel committed enough to succeed.

Muscle balance (pp20-21)

These results will tell you more about the strong (tight) and weak (long) muscles in your body, thus allowing you to develop your own muscle balance and resistance training programme. (*See* Chapter Four, pages 56–59 for explanations of where all the muscles are.)

Question 1 (pelvis):

Neutral – this is a good position to be in, since the spine functions optimally from neutral alignment.
Anterior tilt – generally speaking, this type of pelvic position tends to lead to weak abdominal muscles, tight hip flexors and quadriceps, as well as tight back extensors and weak gluteals and hamstrings.
Posterior tilt– generally speaking, this type of pelvic position tends to lead to tight rectus abdominus muscles (the most superficial abdominal muscles), weak hip flexors and quadriceps, as well as strong hamstrings and weak back extensors and gluteals.
Lopsided tilt – this could mean that you have scoliosis (lateral or sideways curvature) of the spine, that one leg is shorter than the other, or that you have a measure of torso rotation. Visit a back-care practitioner for an accurate diagnosis should your pelvis indicate this position.

Question 2 (legs and feet):

Facing forward – your legs and feet appear to be in a neutral position.
Externally rotated – this tends to indicate strong external hip rotators, so you may wish to include some stretching for them in your programme (*see* 'foot over knee stretch', page 97).
Internally rotated – this tends to indicate strong internal hip rotators, and so including some stretching for them in your programme may help (*see* 'butterfly stretch', page 98).

Question 3 (ankles):

Roll inward – this may indicate weakness in the muscles that stabilize the leg (outer upper leg muscles and hip rotators) and/or tightness in the outer lower leg muscles, and weakness of the opposing muscles (as with the forearm and hand muscles, lower leg and foot muscles are not covered within the scope of this book). Rolling the ankle inwardly, called pronation or eversion, while running or walking can lead to other postural problems, which can often be temporarily eased by orthotics. See a podiatrist if this is a concern for you, but make sure you also address the muscle imbalances that led to this problem in the first place.
Roll outward – this may be a cause of tight inner lower leg muscles, which are responsible for rolling the foot outwards (called supination or inversion), coupled with a weakness in the opposing muscles. Again, since this imbalance can cause problems with a running or walking gait, seek the help of a specialist for diagnosis and treatment.

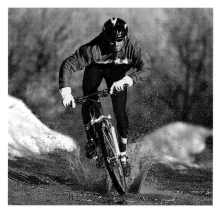
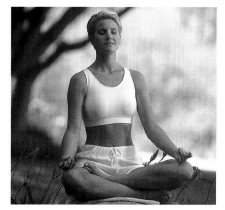
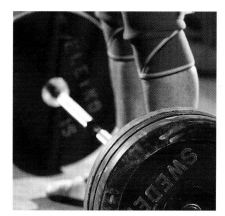

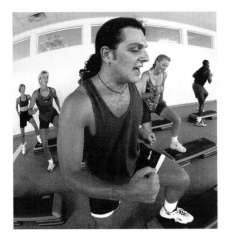

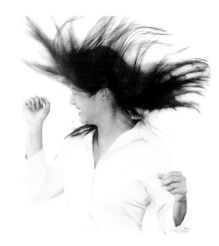

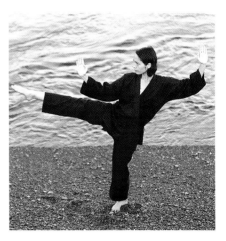

Question 4 (knees):

Inward – this can indicate a weakness in the muscles that stabilize the leg (outer upper leg muscles and hip rotators). Include exercises that strengthen these muscles.
Outward – this may indicate that you have strong external hip rotators, so you may wish to include some stretching for them in your programme (*see* 'foot over knee stretch', page 97).

Question 5 (arms and hands):

Neutral position – this indicates no major imbalances.
Externally rotated – this may relate to tight posterior rotator cuff (shoulder stabilizers) and shoulder muscles. Since many upper body exercises that internally rotate the arm are described in Chapter Four, you should be able to counter these tight muscles fairly effectively.
Internally rotated – this is a far more common imbalance than the one above, due to the fact that so many of the upper body muscles perform this action. Try to include the 'external arm rotator' exercise (*see* page 72) to help to rebalance the arms.

Question 6 (shoulders):

Drooping forward – this may indicate tightness in the chest muscles, coupled with strong internal rotators of the shoulder (many of the back muscles have this function). There may also be weakness in the serratus anterior muscle (*see* the 'reading pose' exercise, page 63), responsible for holding the shoulder blades flat against the back and thus pulling the shoulders backwards.
Rolling backward – tightness in the back muscles, coupled with a weakness in the chest muscles may cause this imbalance. Look for some back stretches and chest strengtheners in Chapter Four.
Lopsided – this is an indication that a muscle or group of muscles on one side of the body is tighter than its counterparts on the opposite side of the body. Since – given the scope of this book – it would be difficult for you to determine just which muscles are responsible for this imbalance, it would be better to seek the help of a practitioner who has specialist knowledge in the area of muscle balance.

Question 7 (upper back):

Rounded – the same issues may exist as with the drooping forward shoulders, so apply the same advice. The term for this curvature is kyphosis. You would probably also benefit from doing the 'thoracic release' on page 94.
Straight – although the back should not be ramrod straight, if your upper back appears to be fairly upright, this is generally a sign that no major imbalances exist in this area. Having said this, though, you would probably still benefit from torso stabilization work (see the torso stabilization section on page 60).

Question 8 (ears):

In front of – this suggests you may be keeping your neck in a habitually extended position, which means that the muscles responsible for keeping the head up are overworked and thus overly strong. Make an effort to pull your chin in while keeping it parallel to the floor and push the back of your neck backwards so your neck is lengthened and not excessively curved.

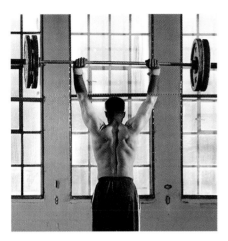

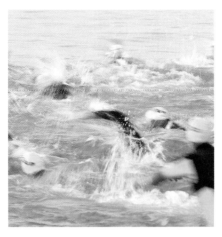

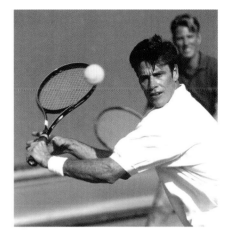

In line with – it would appear that no major imbalances are present in this area.

Question 9 (shoulder blades):

Stick out – this could indicate tightness in the muscles between the shoulder blades (rhomboids, trapezuis). Look for relevant back stretches in Chapter Four, and try to incorporate both the 'hitcher' and 'reading' exercises on pages 62 and 63 to strengthen the muscles, which have an opposing action.
Are flat against – it would appear that no major imbalances are present in this area.

Question 10 (knees):

Behind – you may have swayback legs, which have a tendency to overlock when straightened. This can throw your pelvis into a position other than neutral. Try to avoid fully straightening your knees when you are standing or walking; concentrate instead on controlling your knee extension with the muscles of your thighs.
In line with – this is an optimal position for the legs to be in, in relation to the pelvis.

Exercise preference (p23)

Question 1 relates to cardiovascular activities of a moderate to high intensity, such as walking, running, cycling, swimming, hiking, roller-blading, ice skating, cross-country skiing, sand-boarding and snow-boarding.

Question 2 relates to resistance training, which requires you to strengthen your muscles through the use of a resistance or load. This covers training for muscle balance (*see* the torso stabilization section on page 60), muscle strength or muscle endurance (*see* resistance training, page 67).

Question 3 relates to activities that work your joint range of motion, such as stretch classes, Pilates or yoga.

Question 4 could include most dance activities, such as ballet, ballroom, Latin American, hip-hop, contemporary, etc. If you like the idea of challenging your body to perform set, patterned, rhythmic movements that require skill, co-ordination and mental alertness, then these types of activities are for you.

Question 5 relates to any group activity – for example, a formally structured exercise class – that uses music phrasing for effect, such as indoor cycling, step, low impact, high impact, toning, etc. Exercising to music can help to pass the time and can be quite fun – especially if you sing along.

Question 6 relates to activities that must be learned and practised because skills are required for effective workout completion. These include Capoeira (a currently popular fight form), T'ai Chi, karate, kickboxing, boxing and martial arts-based fitness classes.

Question 7 concerns any activity that can be done effectively on your own, in other words non-team activities. Many people prefer to be on their own when working out, especially those who dislike the idea of a busy gym or a large running group, for example.

Question 8 concerns activities that can be done in a team or group. Working out as part of a group of exercisers can be highly motivating and good fun. It also lends itself to social interaction, which can often in itself be a reason to get someone exercising.

Question 9 concerns whether or not you are at risk of becoming bored with the same activity again and again. While some people feel comfortable and, in fact, secure with repetition, others feel it may threaten motivation and minimize adherence.

Question 10 is the opposite of Question 9, in that it relates to a desire for people to change the mode of exercise they are using in order to alleviate boredom and include a cross-training component into their programme to challenge the body to adapt to various activities. Cross training can be an excellent way to improve fitness more rapidly.

Question 11 relates to activities requiring explosive power, including racquet sports such as tennis and squash, as well as volleyball, soccer, hockey, rugby, etc. This type of activity requires a fair degree of fitness, since the heart is required to deal with varying – and sometimes extreme – effort levels and heart rates.

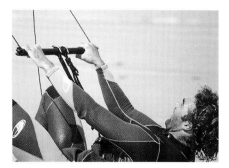
Try outdoor activities for a different and exciting way to achieve fitness.

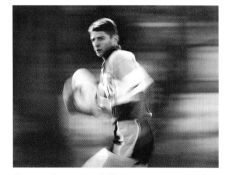
Fast-moving team ball sports are a good way to ensure a hard workout.

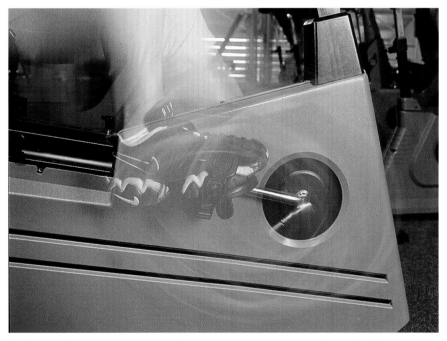
Cycling – either in the gym or on the road – can increase your fitness significantly.

Cardiovascular fitness (p23)

Check your cardiovascular fitness by comparing your results against the scores in the table opposite. If you want to become active on three or more days a week and intend including cardiovascular activities in these sessions, retest yourself after an initial six to eight weeks, and then perhaps every two months or so thereafter. To keep your finger on the pulse of your programme, do not wait for too long between tests. If you are doing really well, it will motivate you to continue; if you discover your fitness has dropped off, it gives you the opportunity to reassess your programme, effort or motivation.

Walk 2.5km (1.5 miles) and check your timing (in minutes) in the table below

FEMALES

Age	20–29	30–39	40–49	50–59	60–69	70–79
E	below 11.47	below 12.50	below 13.35	below 14.54	below 15.56	below 16.43
G	11.48–13.22	12.51–14.23	13.36–14.57	14.55–16.12	15.57–17.06	16.44–18.00
F	13.23–14.49	14.24–15.25	14.58–16.12	16.13–17.14	17.07–18.00	18.01–18.59
P	14.50–16.11	15.26–16.48	16.13–17.29	17.15–18.23	18.01–19.02	19.00–19.56
VP	16.12–19.25	16.49–19.23	17.30–20.04	18.24–20.35	19.03–21.00	19.57–21.36

MALES

Age	20–29	30–39	40–49	50–59	60–69	70–79
E	below 9.14	below 10.01	below 10.47	below 12.01	below 13.22	below 14.37
G	9.15–11.10	10.02–11.39	10.48–12.20	12.02–13.47	13.23–14.59	14.38–16.27
F	11.11–12.25	11.40–12.51	12.21–13.46	13.48–14.54	15.00–16.16	16.28–17.29
P	12.26–13.53	12.52–14.23	13.47–15.07	14.55–16.22	16.17–17.41	17.30–19.02
VP	13.54–18.00	14.24–18.00	15.08–18.31	16.23–19.53	17.42–20.51	19.03–21.05`

E = Well done on an excellent fitness level

G = Your fitness level is good

F = Your fitness level is fair

P = Your fitness level is poor

VP = There is lots of room for improving your fitness level – and you can only get better from here on.

Source: Kenneth Cooper Aerobic Institute

Body composition (p23)

Body Mass Index (BMI):

	Men	Women
Normal	24–27	23–26
Moderately obese	28–31	27–32
Severely obese	> 31	> 32

Source: American College of Sports Medicine

Waist circumference:

Men	Women
• over 94cm (37in) poses an increased risk	• over 80cm (31½ in) poses an increased risk
• over 102cm (40in) poses a high risk	• over 88cm (34½ in) poses a high risk

Source: Exercise Teachers Academy

Planning your
programme

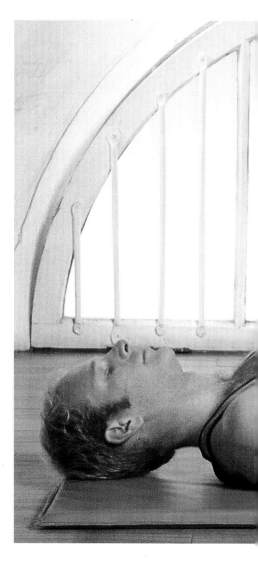

Based on the results of your assessments in Chapter Two, use the information offered here to design your physical activity programme. This section is divided into four main parts – *torso stabilization, resistance training, flexibility training* and *cardiovascular training*. When resistance training is mentioned in the future, this automatically also includes torso stabilization since this form of training uses resistance to challenge the body.

It would be ideal to include a little of each of the four types of training methods described above into any exercise programme, but in the interests of reality, try to choose the types of activities that most fulfil your needs.

Before you begin

There are three components to any workout: warm-up, workout and cool-down. Be sure to follow the advice given for each of these components in order to maximize the effectiveness of your training and minimize the risk of injury.

Warm-up

This prepares your body for the physical activity ahead by increasing the blood supply to working muscles. Begin at a low intensity, slowly increasing intensity over a period of seven to 10 minutes. You should literally feel warm by the end of this period, but definitely not out of breath. Ideally, a warm-up should mimic the movements you are about to do in your workout. For example, if you will be running, try a walk or a light jog. If, however, you will be swimming, complete a few slow, leisurely laps. The idea is that the muscles to be targeted in the workout are the ones that you should try to use in your warm-up.

Whether or not you stretch after your warm-up is entirely up to you. A guideline would be to look at your chosen workout: if you intend doing a kickboxing class, then you should stretch before your workout; if, however, you are about to go for a walk or run, it may not be necessary to include stretching beforehand.

Workout

This relates to the main component of your physical activity programme – it could be cardiovascular, resistance or flexibility training.

Cool-down

This should be completed once you have finished your workout. It entails slowly bringing your heart rate and breathing back to normal.

Ideally, you should dedicate at least five minutes to your cool-down, followed by some post-workout stretching to reduce the effects of stiffness, especially if you have worked on muscles you do not ordinarily use. You could also extend your cool-down period to include relaxation techniques such as deep breathing or meditation. This is a good way to prepare your-

self for the day ahead or end your day with some stress management. It can also provide benefits, such as reduced blood pressure and muscle tension, a positive effect on brain-waves and nerves, and eventually a stronger immune system.

How do you exercise effectively?

Whether you are engaging in resistance, flexibility or cardiovascular training, you need to adhere to some general principles. The first of these is the principle of *overload*, which states that the body must be stimulated beyond its current ability to elicit an adaptation or response. The stimulus is thus the overload.

Other principles include *frequency, intensity, type* and *time* (FITT), *progression, specificity* and *reversibility*. These apply to all methods of training, but here is an example using cardiovascular training.

You have been walking your dog most days of the week for 30 minutes at a time. During this walk, you are not out of breath, nor do you sweat or feel as though you are exerting yourself in any way. You want to increase your fitness level using this time you have put aside for dog walking.

By exercising more regularly, you increase the *frequency* of your

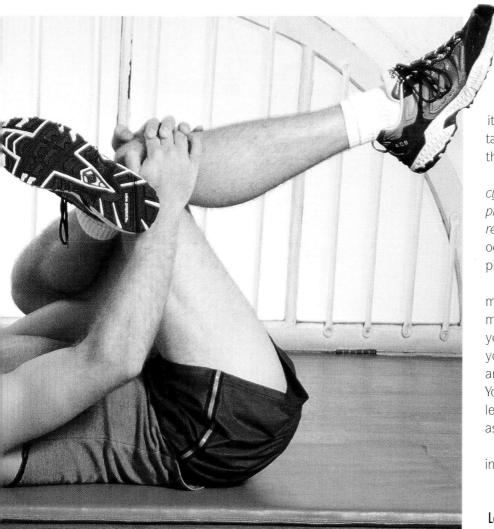

Left: A foot-over-knee stretch helps to improve flexibility in the buttocks and legs.

physical activity. As you have been walking the dog on most days of the week, you might choose now to do so every day. Alternatively, you could use the principle of *intensity* and simply walk faster (*see* also Measuring heart rate, page 103). Yet another way to challenge your body would be to change the *type* of exercise; you could jog, cycle or roller-blade with the dog in tow.

Another of the FITT training variables relates to the amount of *time* spent exercising in a particular session. In this case you have been using 30 minutes for your physical activity. If you do not want to increase the length of your workout, you need to adjust the other three variables, but if you are prepared to increase the duration of your exercise session, you can keep the other variables as they were.

Bear in mind that changing more than one variable at once brings about new options. For example, you could actually shorten your workout time and perform an activity requiring more intense effort. Or you could exercise less frequently but for a longer time at the same intensity as before.

The principle of *progression* refers to the fact that to see improvements you need to constantly adapt your programme to challenge your body. In essence, this means that your programme will become harder and harder.

A guideline would be as follows:
Beginners (weeks 1–6): three times a week, increasing to three or four times; duration from 15 minutes, increasing to 30 minutes; cardio intensity from 55 per cent,

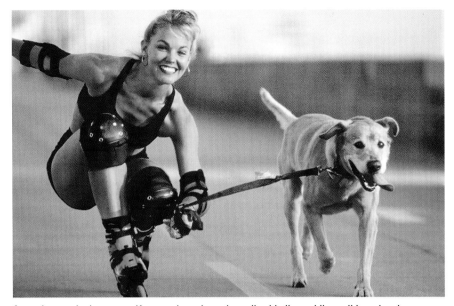

Save time and give yourself a good workout by roller-blading while walking the dog.

increasing to 70 per cent maximum heart rate (*see* page 103); resistance training geared more towards muscular endurance.
Intermediate (weeks 6–14); five times a week; duration 40 minutes; cardio intensity to 80 per cent maximum heart rate; resistance training can include more muscular strength work.

Specificity relates to the type of exercise you choose. If your goal is to get fit enough to run, for instance, swimming will not achieve this goal; you need to run in order to get running fit. It is always a good idea to start slowly, so a combination of walking and running would be best in this case.

Looking at the principle of *reversibility*, let us assume that you chose to run with the dog. You have been consistent with your programme for four weeks and then are suddenly unable to continue for a short while – perhaps you go on a business trip

for a few weeks. The reversibility principle is: 'use it or lose it'. In other words, if the challenge provided to the body by means of your run is no longer present, the adaptation made by your body may be lost. As a rule, the longer you have been exercising or providing your body with a challenge, the more slowly the results of your body's adaptation will be lost.

As with any physical activity programme, always progress slowly and safely. Start with a shorter duration and lower intensity; if at any stage you feel distressed or in pain, stop exercising immediately and seek professional advice.

As important as all of these training principles, but often overlooked, is the need for rest. Training through fatigue, or training too often at too high an intensity, can result in injury. It can also plateau or even diminish the benefits of your training. Listen to your body and go easy on it when you feel tired.

How can you promote your health?

Using the information in this book, there are two routes you can take to improve health and/or fitness. The first encourages and promotes health, and the second relates to improvements in fitness.

What can you do to promote your health? (The issue of fitness will be dealt with later, *see* page 43.) Since generally accepted guidelines indicate that about 30 minutes of moderate-intensity activity is required daily to achieve this goal, it makes sense to make some lifestyle changes that encourage you to move your body as frequently as possible through the course of your day in order to accumulate this time. You do not need to do all 30 minutes of activity at once; if it helps you remain motivated to exercise, break your sessions up into smaller periods of physical activity.

Here is an example. You start work at 08:00 and are extremely busy behind your desk until lunchtime. You know you have the option to take lunch, but you always work straight through, so that you can complete the tasks on hand. Invariably, you eat a sandwich at your desk, where you remain until 17:00. When you get home, you need to help feed and bath the children, take the dog for a stroll, read the paper and more. You also enjoy the idea of socializing with friends or watching a favourite television programme or movie as a way to unwind. By the time you go to bed you are exhausted. So when do you exercise?

Why not take the dog out in the morning for a 10-minute brisk walk around the block, grab a 10-minute walk at lunchtime just before you eat, and another in the evening with the dog. Not only will the dog be your best friend, you will have accumulated your 30 minutes of health-enhancing physical activity.

Try also to be as active during other parts of the day as possible. Again, this involves making some appropriate behaviour changes to

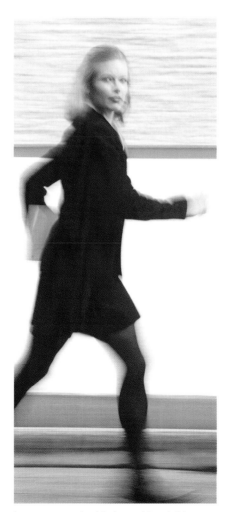

Improve your health by making brisk walking a part of your lunchtime routine.

support a more active lifestyle. Although by now the following suggestions may seem passé – you have probably heard every conceivable fitness or health professional recommend them – they still stand as really helpful ways to keep your metabolism ticking over and reduce the negative effects of inactivity.

- Take the stairs instead of the elevator. Start off gradually by taking the elevator up and walking down until this becomes a habit, then try walking up too. The same applies to escalators.
- When looking for a parking bay, try to find one further away from your destination and walk briskly.
- Walk when talking on your mobile phone, unless of course this affects signal strength.
- Make time for gardening and pool cleaning. If you have neither garden nor pool, ask friends if you can get stuck into theirs – they will not say no.
- If your city has an efficient public transport system, use it as this will invariably require a lot of walking between stations.
- If you need to get a message or document to a colleague at work, or need information from elsewhere in the building, get up and do it yourself rather than sending an SMS, email or messenger.
  Think of any other habitual shortcuts you use to avoid expending energy and try to implement changes. Since they are often entrenched habits, do not be too hard on yourself if you forget and go back to old behaviours from time to time.

In brief

- Always warm up before and cool down after your workout.
- Remember to apply the principles of overload, progression, specificity, reversibility and FITT (that is, frequency, intensity, type and time).
- Begin your programme with shorter duration and lower-intensity exercises.
- For improved health accumulate 30 minutes or more of moderate-intensity physical activity on most, preferably all, days of the week.
- Be sure to remain as active through other parts of your day as possible.

Torso stabilization
What is it?

This type of training deals with torso (trunk) stability. It is really important to address major imbalances in the torso before you adopt any kind of resistance training programme, or at least at the same time, since increasing the strength of a muscle that is already overdeveloped can have far-reaching negative postural consequences.

If you have already completed your own postural assessment (see pages 20–22) you will have a better idea of which areas of your body need to be stretched and/or strengthened. Complete the assessment now if you have not yet done it, so that you can be as specific as possible about this aspect of your training.

Generally speaking, people tend to strengthen those body parts that feel comfortable being worked – namely, the strong muscles. However, it is the muscles that feel as though they are not able to perform as well that should be activated and strengthened. Similarly, people tend to stretch those muscles that feel comfortable being stretched – namely, the already long muscles. It would follow, then, that these are the muscles that should rather be strengthened, while muscles that are uncomfortable when stretched are the very ones that need some flexibility training.

If you have identified in yourself any postural weaknesses or imbalances, or if you simply want to strengthen your torso muscles, include some, if not all, of the exercises covered in Chapter Four under the heading Torso Stabilization (see pages 60–66). This section also includes functional abdominal training rather than traditional abdominal exercises, as functional exercises target the muscles that stabilize the pelvis and help to keep it in neutral, optimal alignment (pictured right).

As you work through the exercises, try to maintain good posture. This can help to improve both your breathing and general movement, and can decrease the risk of injury. Create ways to remind yourself to check your posture through the day and counter the damaging effects of constant sitting by standing or moving frequently. Try to build these exercises into your weekly routine so that you complete them at least two to three times a week.

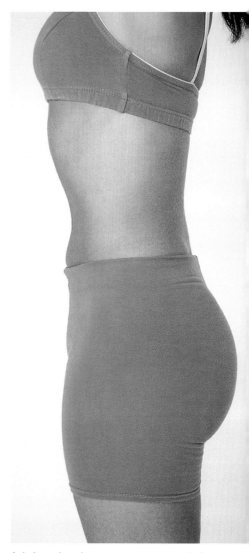

A balanced and strong torso can result in more powerful, effective movement.

Another reason you might choose to strengthen your torso is to help isolate the primary movers, or the main muscles activated, in any given muscle-strengthening exercise. For example, holding the torso completely still in a bicep curl by activating the stabilizers compounds the effect on the biceps due to the fact that they are isolated. If you do not have the strength to use your

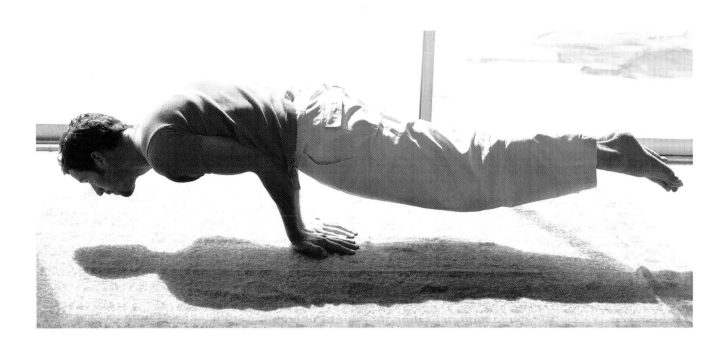

torso stabilizers, the trunk may inadvertently help the biceps through the use of momentum – you may have witnessed someone in a gym using his or her back instead of the arms to swing the weights upwards.

In brief

- Address major torso imbalances before beginning any muscle-building programme.
- Stretch tight muscles and strengthen weak muscles.
- Do more functional abdominal stabilization training.
- Try to attain neutral alignment of the spine.
- Check your posture regularly through the day.

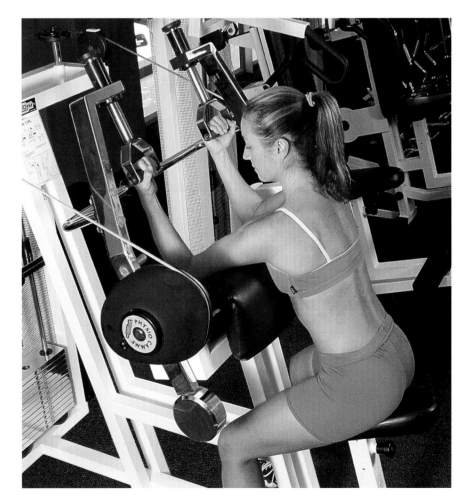

Top: Choose any style of workout that will challenge and motivate you.
Right: Keeping the torso still while using the bicep curl isolates the biceps.

Resistance training
What is it?

Resistance training simply means strengthening a muscle through the use of resistance or a load. Many people know this form of training as toning or muscle building. There are two specific routes you can take when you embark on resistance training, based on your desired outcome.

If your goal is to develop *muscle endurance* – useful for activities like carrying shopping, picking up children and gardening – or if you just want to tone your muscles without building too much size, you need to select a load that allows for the muscle to perform quite a few repetitions (reps) before fatiguing. Due to different body types, people respond uniquely to weight training, but there are general norms that can be applied fairly effectively. For muscle endurance training, perform up to 18 or 20 repetitions at a weight that starts to fatigue you at 14 or 15.

If your goal is more about *building strength* – good for activities like moving a large piece of furniture or picking up a heavy box – or if you want to develop slightly more significant muscle size, perform up to 10 or 12 repetitions at a weight that starts to fatigue you at seven or eight. It is only when you want to develop maximal strength – in other words, the very heaviest a muscle can lift for one repetition – that you would work with a load that allows between one to four or five reps. Body builders and power lifters tend to train at this level.

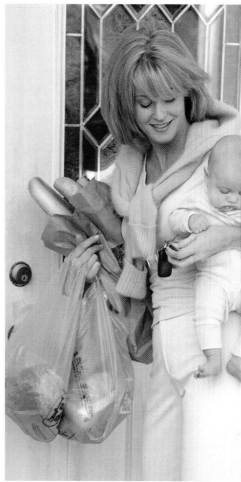

Right: Resistance training helps to build muscle endurance to cope with daily tasks.

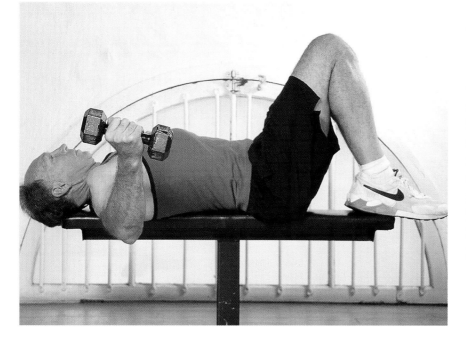

Why should you do it?

Everyone is aware of the aesthetic benefits of toned muscles. Some other reasons you might want to engage in this type of training include better management of stress, improved athletic performance, a reduction in the effects of ageing, prevention and/or treatment of osteoporosis (decreased bone density), better control of body weight and injury prevention and/or rehabilitation.

Flyes are resistance training exercises that help to strengthen the chest.

How can you make your muscles grow?

To make muscle develop, you must use the principle of overload discussed at the beginning of this chapter (*see* page 31). For your muscles to increase their strength, they need to be challenged by a load.

There are a few ways you can provide this challenge within the context of resistance training. For example, if you can currently perform five press-ups without too much effort and your goal is to strengthen your chest and tricep muscles, one way that you could overload these muscles is to do more than five repetitions. You may find that by the eighth one, you are really battling and so you stop. You have placed an overload on the relevant muscles, simply by adding three more repetitions.

You could also choose to do two or more sets of the same exercise, or you could reduce your recovery time between sets.

A final method for increasing overload in this example would be to place your feet up on a step so that you add more resistance to the exercise. By lifting your feet, you shift more body weight forward into the arms, making the exercise harder for the targeted muscles. When using this last method to challenge the body, increase your load gradually and by no more than 5 per cent at a time. This is easy enough when working with weighted equipment, but a little hard to gauge with a body-weight exercise; in this case, let comfort be your guide.

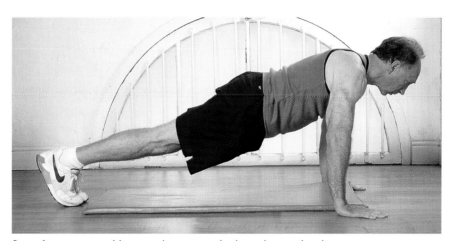

Do a few extra repetitions to place an overload on the muscles that you want to grow.

How many sets?

The example above raises the question of how many sets (groups of repetitions) to do for any given exercise. There are varied opinions about this issue; try to find a system that works for you and your chosen lifestyle. While it is true that you gain muscular benefit from doing two or more sets, and some people do as many as five, it is also true that if you execute single-set resistance exercises with concentration, focus and good form – that is, without using momentum – you will see similar benefits. The single-set option is a good one for people with time constraints, or for those who just do not want to spend too much time training.

If you choose to do more than one set per exercise, you have two options. The first is to perform the sets one after the other, with a short recovery period in between. Recovery can range from 30 seconds to a few minutes, depending on the intensity with which you are training. The second option is to perform one set of one type of

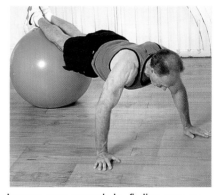

Improve your strength by finding ways to challenge the muscles targeted.

exercise, such as a press-up, and then another set of a different type of exercise, such as a squat, so that you give the first group of muscles a rest while working another. You would then go back to the first exercise and repeat the process. This is known as active recovery and is, once again, a great time saver.

How many exercises?

Another issue you need to address is the number of exercises chosen per body part, per training session. You will notice in the Exercise

Menu in Chapter Four that some exercises significantly target other muscles as well as the main muscle/s. These are called *compound exercises*, which kill two or more birds with one stone, so to speak. They are excellent if you are short of time as they cut down training time considerably. The fact that they target more than one muscle at once also means they are more functional, since most of our daily movements entail using groups of muscles at any one time.

Other exercises are noted as *isolation exercises*, and are therefore very specific to the main muscle being worked. These are good for adding variety to your programme and for specific strength gains, although training one particular muscle group more than others may lead to imbalances and possibly injury, so be sure to balance out your isolation exercises.

Look at the results of your posture assessment (*see* pages 20–22) before deciding which and how many exercises per body part to include in your resistance programme, since the goal is to develop a muscularly balanced body. Try to select at least one compound exercise from each of the body-part categories noted in Chapter Four (*see* pages 67–68). Even better would be to select exercises based on the main muscle/s used, thus ensuring efficiency and balance. For example, if you choose press-ups as a chest and tricep exercise, concentrate on the biceps and omit the triceps when you choose your arm exercises, as you have worked them in the press-up.

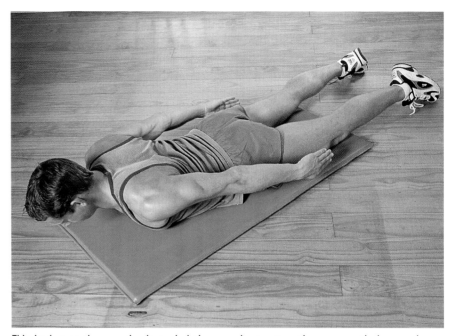

This back extension exercise is an isolation exercise to strengthen one particular muscle.

How often?

For optimal strength gains try to complete your chosen routine at least three times a week. If you are hard-pressed for time, however, twice a week should be enough for maintenance, provided that you are employing appropriate concentration and good form. Resistance training just once a week will provide few benefits. Remember that the principle of overload applies here too – challenge the body enough to force it to adapt.

Depending on how much time you have available to devote to a resistance training programme, you could choose to do either a *standard routine* (which uses the same body parts each time you train), or a *split routine* (which uses different body parts on different days).

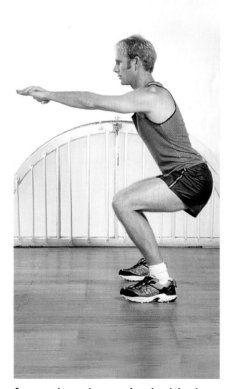

Compound exercises are functional in that they mimic natural movements.

An example of a STANDARD RESISTANCE training routine for the upper body might be:

2 x sets push-ups (main muscles: chest and triceps)

1 x set overhead arm extensions (main muscle: triceps)

2 x sets latissimus (lat) pulldowns (main muscles: back and biceps)

1 x set bicep curls (main muscle: bicep group)

1 x set side raises (main muscle: deltoids)

1 x set front raises (main muscle: deltoids)

An example of a SPLIT ROUTINE might be:

Day one: chest and triceps

2 x sets push-ups (main muscles: chest and triceps)

1 x set overhead arm extensions (main muscle: triceps)

2 x sets flyes, i.e. arms opening and closing above the chest, dumbbells in hand (main muscle: chest)

Day two: back, shoulders and biceps

2 x sets lat pulldowns (main muscles: back and biceps)

1 x set bicep curls (main muscle: bicep group)

1 x set side raises (main muscle: deltoids)

1 x set front raises (main muscle: deltoids)

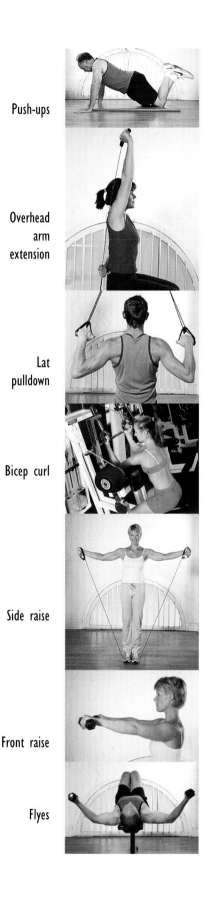

Push-ups

Overhead arm extension

Lat pulldown

Bicep curl

Side raise

Front raise

Flyes

Note that the compound exercise/s of any chosen muscle group precede the isolation exercise/s. This ensures that you retain full strength on the more functional of the two exercises, and reduces the risk of injury. If you feel fatigued during the isolation exercise, simply reduce the amount of weight you are using.

Choosing a split routine means that you will be exercising twice as often as you would be if you were using a standard routine. However, you will generally be working out for longer with a standard routine, since you need to work the whole body rather than just half of it. Whichever you choose, try to give your muscles approximately 48 hours of rest between workouts.

What equipment should you use?

Some of the exercises covered in Chapter Four do not utilize any form of external load. Instead, they are *body-weight exercises*, which will facilitate an increase in muscle size proportionate to your body. With these exercises, perform as many repetitions as you can while keeping good form and technique.

The Exercise Menu in Chapter Four also includes some exercises you can use if you have access to the *equipment* required. Do not worry if you do not – a couple of different exercises are given for each muscle group, allowing you some flexibility when making your choices. Where you see the need to use weights and you do not

have access to these, simply substitute with water bottles filled with sand or water, or sandbags. If you are using gym equipment for your training, you will probably have the option of using either *free weights* or *machines*. Machines are often best for beginners, as there is less chance of injury and minimal skill is required to perform the exercise effectively. Once you feel comfortable enough with your skill level, it is a good idea to start including some free weights into your programme, since this mode of training is definitely more functional. In other words, it allows the body to move naturally through the execution of the exercise, whereas machines tend to place you in one position and restrict you to that position throughout.

In brief

- For muscle endurance – 18 to 20 reps, starting to fatigue at 14 to 15 reps.
- For building strength – 10 to 12 reps, starting to fatigue at seven to eight reps.
- Single sets are effective if you apply concentration and good form during execution.
- If performing more than one set, do them one after the other, with short recovery periods (30 seconds to a few minutes). Alternatively, do one set of one type of exercise and then another set of a different type of exercise, repeating this cycle.
- Use compound exercises for more functional exercises and to target more than one muscle at a time.
- Use isolation exercises for variety and for specific strength gains.
- For optimal strength gains complete your chosen routine at least three times per week; if hard-pressed for time, twice a week should suffice.
- Choose either a standard routine (same body parts each time you train), or a split routine (different body parts on different days).

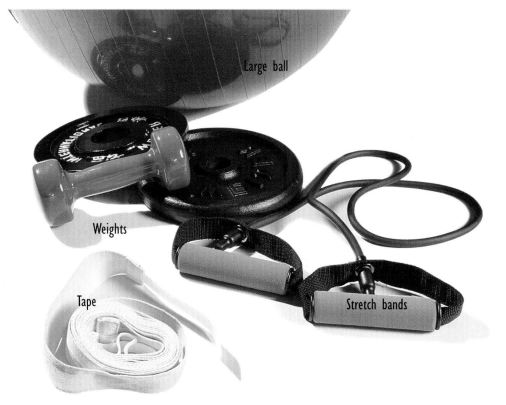

Large ball

Weights

Tape

Stretch bands

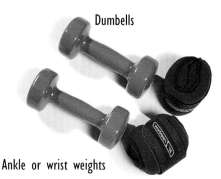

Dumbells

Ankle or wrist weights

Flexibility training
What is it?

The word flexibility refers to the range of motion around a joint. While some people are born more or less flexible than the average person, others may have become more or less flexible through habitual posture, inactivity or over-training in one particular muscle or muscle group. Unless a specific disability or injury exists, it is possible to ensure a full range of motion in all joints through sound and safe flexibility training.

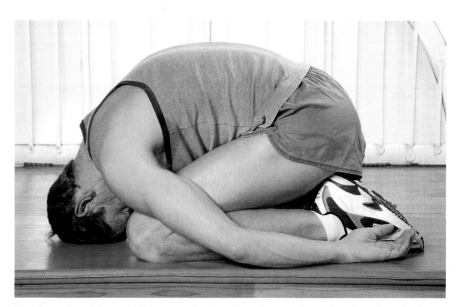

The forward curl is an isolation stretch that allows for complete relaxation of the body.

Why should you do it?

There are a number of reasons why flexibility training is an essential part of any exercise programme. One is that it may reduce the risk of injury, since the act of stretching a muscle that has been worked hard provides release and relief to the tension created by the muscle contraction.

Another reason is that it ensures postural balance. For example, people who are excessively developed in their chest may end up with both their arms and shoulders drooping forward, giving them a stance that resembles that of a primate. In this case, further developing the chest without stretching it will only exacerbate the postural imbalance. First prize would be to strengthen the back and stretch the chest until such time as back strength matches chest strength.

Yet another reason is increased range of motion, which could lead to an improvement in co-ordination. Other benefits may include decreased post-exercise muscle soreness, as well as improved body awareness, increased muscle relaxation and improved circulation.

As with other forms of training, you need to build up this aspect of fitness over time. Be aware, though, that improving your flexibility is a much slower process than that of increasing strength and cardiovascular fitness. It requires considerably more dedication and commitment, but is well worth the effort.

When should you do it?

If you are using flexibility training as part of a greater training programme, it would be advisable to leave it till last, since your goal is to stretch muscles that are either habitually tight, or those that have just been used in your training programme. If you are using only flexibility training as

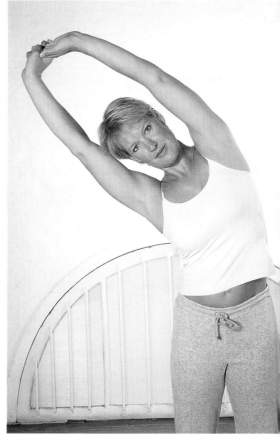

The standing side stretch is a compound exercise that helps to improve flexibility.

your chosen programme, be sure to warm up your body before attempting to stretch, since warm muscles respond more effectively than cold ones. Some stretches may feel very uncomfortable to you. As long as you do not feel pain, try to stay with the stretch, even if for a few seconds initially. Do not bounce while stretching and be sure to breathe through-out a stretch – the more relaxed your body is, the easier it will feel and the deeper you will be able to take the stretch. Stretching at odd times through the day – while at work, while watching television or while reading – can also be beneficial if carried out with awareness and good form. Stretching after sitting or standing for long periods can help prevent the discomfort associated with lack of movement.

How should you do it?

It is vital for you to maintain correct alignment during your stretches. Stretches are listed and described in Chapter Four, with relevant cues for good technique, so try to follow these. Many of the stretches covered are *compound stretches* – that is, they deal with more than one muscle at the same time – while others are *isolation stretches*. The compound stretches are great time savers, whereas the isolation stretches are very specif-ic and may be better for you if you know you have an issue with a particular muscle group that needs to be stretched – for example, your hamstrings.

How long should you hold it?

A general recommendation for increasing muscle length and initiating a relaxation response in the same muscle is that a stretch should be held for between 30 and 90 seconds, and it should be performed two to three times per week. This is not to say, however, that stretching every day would have negative side effects; in fact, it would be very beneficial if you are using it to help to counter postural tightness.

In brief

- If using flexibility training as part of a greater programme, leave it till after your workout.
- If using only flexibility training as your chosen programme, warm up before you start.
- Do not bounce while stretching and be sure to breathe.
- Maintain correct body alignment during your stretches.
- Do not stretch through pain.
- Hold stretches for between 30 and 90 seconds.
- Stretching can be done daily.

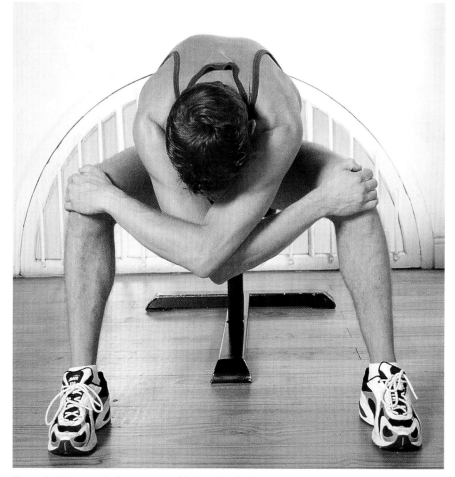

If you hold a stretch for a reasonable length of time, you will feel the tension ease out of the area that is being stretched.

Cardiovascular training
What is it?

According to the Exercise Teachers Academy, 'the term *cardiovascular* or *aerobic* exercise generally refers to a form of exercise that is long in duration, utilizes the systems of the body in a compound manner, and is performed continuously at an elevated heart rate.'

Why should you do it?

As with resistance and flexibility training, cardiovascular exercise plays an important part in developing overall health and fitness. Many people are aware of the beneficial role that this type of activity plays in weight maintenance, and since obesity and being overweight are on the increase globally, it is appropriate that you understand its role. However, there are definitely times when cardiovascular activity – particularly of a high intensity – is not appropriate. It is absolutely imperative for people who either present a number of risk factors for lifestyle diseases (*see* screening assessment on page 17), or who have been diagnosed with such a disease, to gain medical clearance before starting any exercise programme.

The following list, adapted from the American College of Sports Medicine's cardiorespiratory guidelines, shows the benefits you may experience from increasing your cardiovascular fitness:

- Decreased fatigue in daily activities
- Improved work, recreational, and sports performance

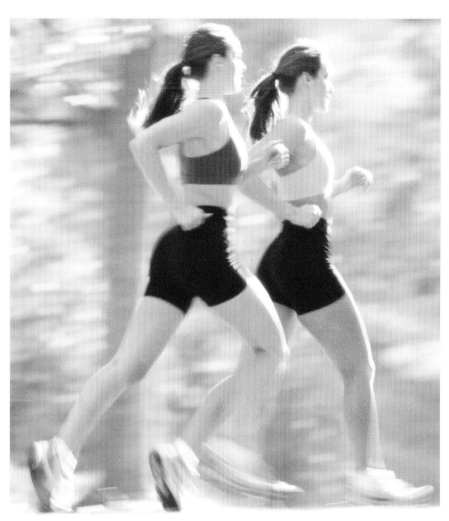

Cardiovascular exercise decreases risk of disease and improves immune system function.

- Decreased risk of:
  Mortality from all causes
  Coronary artery disease
  Cancer (colon, breast)
  Hypertension (high blood pressure)
  Non-insulin-dependent diabetes
  Osteoporosis
  Anxiety
  Depression
- Improved blood fat profile
- Improved immune system function
- Improved glucose tolerance

(glucose, the end product of digested carbohydrates, enters the bloodstream and is used by the body as fuel)
- Improved insulin sensitivity (insulin is a hormone released by the body to stabilize blood sugar/glucose levels)
- Improved body composition (lean muscle mass versus fat mass)
- Enhanced sense of wellbeing
- Reduced blood pressure at various work rates

What is your goal?

One of the most important issues you need to address when looking at developing your own cardio-vascular training programme is whether you wish simply to *improve your health*, or to *become fit*.

These are different concepts: you can train to become healthy, but not necessarily increase your fitness level. Which you choose will depend on the goals you set yourself with regard to your physical activity programme. The American College of Sports Medicine and the Center for Disease Control and Prevention developed a joint statement that concludes: 'Every US adult should accumulate 30 minutes or more of moderate-intensity physical activity on most, preferably all, days of the week.' This statement refers to the *basic health benefits* related to cardiovascular activity (*see* How can you promote your health? on page 33). For improvements in *fitness*, exercise intensity needs to be higher.

How much, how often, how hard?

This brings us to the issue of measuring exercise intensity. The outcome of the measurement will allow you to better understand how your heart is coping with the activity being performed, as well as how its strength is improving over the course of your programme. *See* page 103 for details on monitoring heart rate and fitness.

This section offers guidelines you can use to develop your fitness-related cardiovascular programme. This type of programme is more formal and structured and requires greater commitment, motivation and energy than a programme dealing only with health promotion, but its rewards are commensurately greater.

Having completed the assessments in Chapter Two, you may have established that you want to achieve very specific goals. Use the information below as the basis for your programme, but bear in mind that you are a unique individual and may respond to and be comfortable with a different approach. Use yourself as a guinea pig and experiment with different variables to find out what works best for you. (*See* How do you exercise effectively? on page 31.)

While exercising every day is ideal, exercising that many times at a high intensity is not. Try to

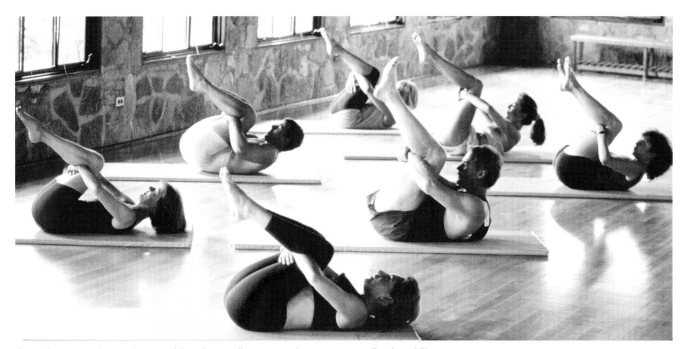

Exercising to music can be a useful and rewarding way to learn new co-ordination skills.

vary your workouts so that intensity levels change from day to day. For example, you may be looking to lose some excess body fat and become a little fitter. You are prepared to put in 40 minutes every day, except Sunday, when you would prefer to take a day off or just to go for a pleasant stroll in a forest, along the beach or in the mountains.

A recommended *six-day programme* would look something like the one in the box below:

SIX-DAY PROGRAMME
(for intermediate to advanced)

MONDAY:
40-minute high-intensity indoor cycling class at the local gym
TUESDAY:
20 minutes of moderate-intensity running, followed by 20 minutes of resistance training and stretching
WEDNESDAY:
30-minute high-intensity mix of stationary cycling, treadmill running and stepping, followed by a 10-minute stretch
THURSDAY:
as for Tuesday
FRIDAY:
as for Monday
SATURDAY:
20-minute moderate-intensity swim, followed by 20 minutes of resistance training

---

What if you can only put in one hour, three times a week? A recommended *three-day programme* would look something like this:

THREE -DAY PROGRAMME

MONDAY:
40-minute high-intensity indoor cycling class at the local gym, followed by 15 minutes of resistance training and five minutes of stretching
WEDNESDAY:
35-minute high-intensity mix of stationary cycling, treadmill running and stepping, followed by 15 minutes of resistance training and 10 minutes of stretching
FRIDAY:
as for Monday

Notice that all three are high-intensity workouts. This is simply because any other activity done during the day or week will more than likely be moderate or low-intensity in nature.

If you find you are getting bored with your cardiovascular work, you could choose to perform shorter periods interspersed with resistance training — for example, 2 x 15 minutes of cycling, followed by 10 minutes of resistance training. Bear in mind, though, that if your goal is to get fit rather than to shed excess body fat, you need to

challenge the body's endurance capacity or its ability to perform continuous aerobic activity over an extended period.

A word of caution to those who choose to exercise for fitness: adopt the recommendations for a lifestyle change made to those who choose to be active for health benefits only (*see* page 33). All too often, exercisers become inactive through the rest of their day, believing that in the time put aside for structured exercise they have done all that is required in terms of energy expenditure and movement. As a result, their fitness programme does not actually support a holistic approach to an active lifestyle. You should not become too reliant on your structured exercise time for improved health, as there may be times when you cannot complete these sessions because of illness, injury or travel, and would therefore benefit greatly from other methods of activity.

What type of activity should you choose?

Choosing an aerobic activity you feel comfortable with may require you to experience a number of different modes before settling for the best of a few options. Remember, you want to provide ways of challenging the body, as well as reducing the risk of boredom, so always keep a couple of options open.

You may choose to do *weight-bearing exercises* – such as running or walking – during which your body's weight acts against

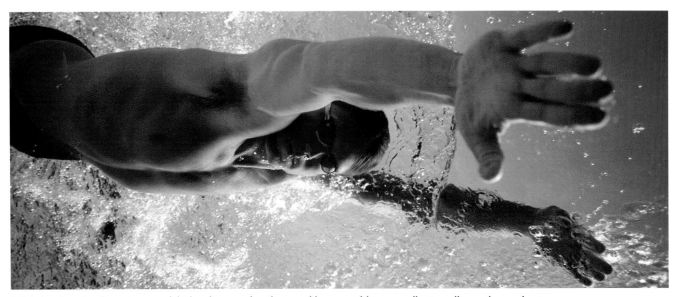

Swimming is a low-impact, non-weight-bearing exercise that provides you with an excellent cardiovascular workout.

gravity, or *non-weight-bearing exercises* — such as swimming or cycling — during which your body's weight against gravity is reduced. If you are overweight or have joint or bone limitations, it may be advisable to choose the non-weight-bearing option, since you will still experience the same benefits without putting yourself at further risk of injury.

If you are suffering from or at risk of developing osteoporosis, weight-bearing activities may be more beneficial than non-weight-bearing activities. This is due to the fact that higher loading on the bones helps to build higher bone density. This is not to suggest that non-weight-bearing activities should be omitted, rather that although you may enjoy these types of activities more, it would be better to include some weight-bearing exercises in your programme.

Give some thought to whether you want to perform *high-impact* (both feet off the ground at a given point) or *low-impact* (one foot always in contact with the ground) activities. These terms refer to the amount of impact the skeletal system experiences during the chosen activity.

See the table below for examples of different types of exercises.

How should you train?

There are a number of different ways you can train, including continuous, interval or fartlek training.

Continuous training refers to cardiovascular activity that remains constant in effort. It is a good way to begin any cardiovascular programme as it allows you to establish a base level of fitness from which you can further challenge the body.

HIGH IMPACT	LOW IMPACT WEIGHT-BEARING	LOW IMPACT NON-WEIGHT-BEARING
• running/jogging • volleyball • gymnastic dance • high-impact aerobic dance • classical and modern dance • most on-land ball sports	• walking • surfing • roller blading/ ice skating • low-impact aerobic dance • ballroom dancing • water-/snow-skiing	• water sports (in which you are suspended) • cycling • swimming • synchronized swimming • rowing

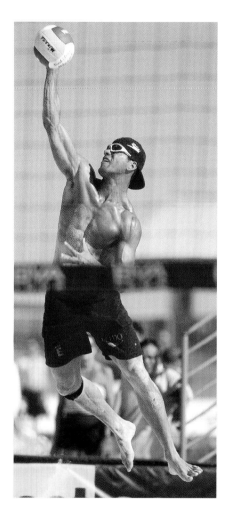

Interval training refers to repetitive, usually measured, cycles of rest and effort – for example, a one-minute sprint, followed by a 30-second rest, repeated many times.

Fartlek training is a Swedish expression referring to non-measured or random moments of high- and low-intensity effort. Although tough, it can be quite fun as it is relatively unstructured. It is not really suitable for beginners.

While the continuous mode is appropriate for a slower, safer introduction to cardiovascular exercise and fitness development, both interval and fartlek training are good for those who are time pressured, or who get bored with repetitive activities. They also provide excellent cross training for the heart as they include high-intensity periods, followed by low-intensity recovery, 'forcing' the heart to cope with a broad range of heart rates.

In brief

- Choose between weight-bearing exercises (body weight acts against gravity, such as running), or non-weight-bearing exercises (body weight against gravity is reduced, such as swimming).
- Choose either high-impact activities (such as running) or low-impact activities (such as walking).
- Start your programme with continuous training (constant in effort), bringing in interval (repetitive, measured cycles of rest and effort) or fartlek training (non-measured or random moments of high and low intensity) at a later stage.
- Challenge the heart by doing different activities at different intensities each time you train.

Far left: Volleyball is a high-impact activity. Below: Surfing is a low-impact, weight-bearing form of exercise.

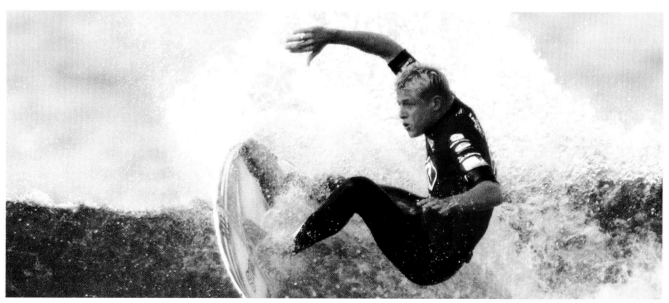

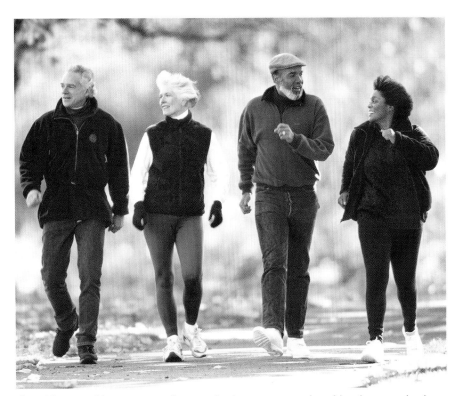

Organizing a walking group can be a motivating way to exercise with other committed exercisers in a social environment.

Special categories
Older adults

Resistance training for older adults is an important part of improving general wellbeing and overall function. As we get older, our tendency is to slow down physically. This happens for a number of reasons. One is that we feel we should. While it is important that you are more careful about acknowledging your limitations as you age, it is equally important that you stay active through your senior years.

Another reason we slow down is that with sedentary living, we become less mobile or more inflexible and thus find it harder to move our bodies through even the simplest of daily activities. This is

one reason why it is so important to include flexibility training in your training programme – at any age.

Resistance training, especially when done against gravity, helps to reduce bone loss, which begins to occur after you pass the age of about 35, when it is at its peak. In this way, you can start to prevent osteoporosis early in life. Resistance training also helps considerably in the management of osteoporosis, since strong muscles can help to share the stress on an affected joint. It has also been shown to slow down bone loss and increase bone density. Increased general strength and stability, which lead to improved balance, may also help prevent fracture injuries from falling.

If you are an 'older adult' – by which we mean someone over 65 years – and you have been sedentary until now, it would not be ideal to do this type of training more than two or three times a week, as the danger of damaging joints may outweigh the nominal benefits of more frequent resistance training. In fact, even if you have been active, a programme that includes resistance training three times a week should be sufficient for maintaining strength. Incorporate a slightly longer warm-up and cool-down period (10 to 15 minutes) and keep your intensity and number of repetitions lower than those suggested for the general population (*see* page 37). Also, use lighter resistance during your first eight weeks or so in order to allow your muscles to respond positively.

When looking to challenge the body, begin by increasing the number of repetitions before increasing the load itself. Stay with weights that allow you a minimum of at least six repetitions, and work within your own joints' range of motion, so you are not working into pain. Pay particular attention to the exercises covered in the torso stabilization section of Chapter Four (*see* page 60), as maintaining good posture becomes even more important with age.

Together with relatively strong muscles and flexible joints, *cardiovascular fitness* also plays an important role in improving overall function and general wellbeing in older adults. Again, if you have been sedentary until now, proceed cautiously with a new programme, allowing your body to respond positively to the new challenge.

As with resistance training, include a longer warm-up and cool-down period and be more aware of personal limitations. These limitations – which may include factors like poor joint mobility or arthritis – will affect the type of activity you choose to engage in. In these cases, non-weight-bearing exercises, such as swimming or cycling, may be preferable to weight-bearing exercise, such as walking or running.

While it is advisable to decrease your training intensity (40 to 65 per cent of maximum heart rate, *see* page 103), it would be beneficial to be active as often as possible (five to seven days per week) for a duration of 20 to 40 minutes. These periods of activity could also be broken up into 15-minute sessions two to three times a day.

Be sure that you get medical clearance before you start an exercise programme so that any health issues that do arise can be dealt with timeously. It is also important to know and understand how healthy your body is so that either your limitations can be acknowledged, or you can feel secure in the knowledge that you are in good health.

Try if possible to make contact with a personal trainer in your area who specializes in training older adults, as you will benefit from working with someone who can offer you a more individualized programme – and therefore a more effective one.

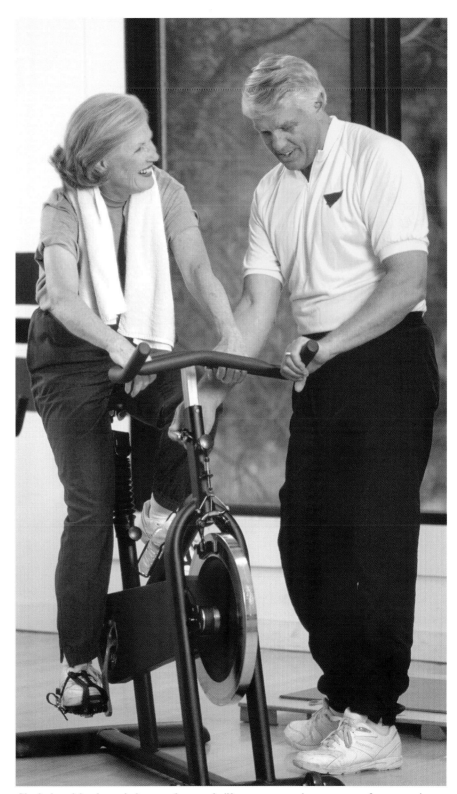

Physical activity is a vital part of anyone's life, no matter what your age. Someone who specializes in training older adults will be able to add value to your programme.

Pregnant women

It is essential to secure medical clearance before starting a physical activity programme. Some contra-indications do exist for exercise during pregnancy (*see right*), but if these do not apply to you and you have been exercising regularly, go ahead and continue to do so. If you have previously been inactive, it is not recommended that you start an exercise programme in the first trimester. Rather wait and begin one slowly in the second trimester.

Resistance training recommendations

This can be a beneficial part of any physical activity programme for pregnant women. By developing stronger muscles, you may help your body to counter postural changes that typically occur during pregnancy. Having said that, however, it is not advisable for all women to resistance-train during pregnancy, as there are a number of contra-indications for exercising during this time. The box on page 51 warns when not to exercise during pregnancy.

General exercise recommendations

Discuss your exercise goals during pregnancy with your doctor and follow these guidelines:

- Do not begin a vigorous exercise programme shortly before or during pregnancy.
- For two reasons, avoid exercising on your back after the first trimester. The first is a reduction in blood flow to the foetus, and the second is the heart's decreased ability to adapt to further demands placed on it, due to an already increased workload.
- Gradually reduce the intensity, duration and frequency of exercise during the second and third trimesters.
- Avoid exercise when humidity and/or temperature is high.
- Try to run or walk on flat, even surfaces.
- Wear supportive shoes while walking or running.
- If running becomes uncomfortable during the second and third trimesters, try other forms of aerobic exercise, such as swimming, running in water and cycling.
- Extend your warm-up and cool-down periods.
- Take your body temperature immediately after exercise. If it exceeds 38°C (10°F), modify intensity and duration, and exercise in cooler conditions.
- Use the rating of perceived exertion scale (*see* page 104) rather than heart rate to monitor exercise intensity. Choose an intensity that is comfortable;

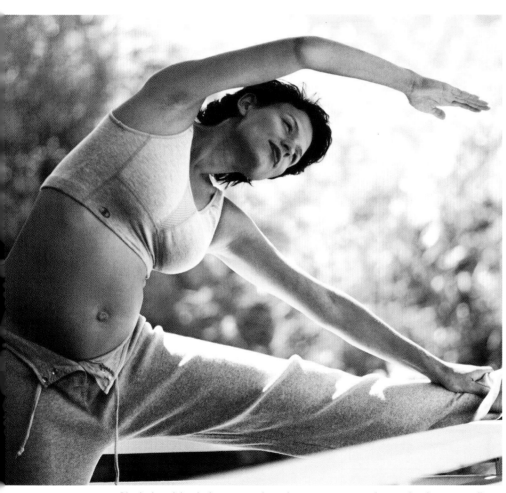

Physical activity is important throughout pregnancy and can also be an excellent form of stress release for moms-to-be.

The American College of Obstetrics and Gynaecology (ACOG) warns of when not to exercise during pregnancy:

1. Pregnancy-induced high blood pressure
2. Pre-term rupture of membrane
3. Pre-term labour during the previous or current pregnancy
4. Incompetent cervix
5. Persistent second to third trimester bleeding
6. Intrauterine growth retardation

Other recommendations from the American College of Sports Medicine for resistance training during pregnancy include:

- Do not participate in resistance training if you have any of the ACOG contra-indications for aerobic exercise during pregnancy (see list above).
- If you have never participated in resistance training do not initiate it during pregnancy.
- Avoid ballistic (bouncing) exercises, as pregnancy is associated with joint and connective tissue laxity, which may increase susceptibility to injury.

- Breathe normally during resistance training, because oxygen delivery to the placenta may be reduced during breath holding.
- Avoid heavy resistance, which may expose the joints, connective tissue and skeletal structures to excessive forces. An exercise set consisting of at least 12–15 repetitions, without unusual fatigue, generally ensures that the resistance is appropriate.
- As you train, overload initially by increasing the number of repetitions and later by increasing resistance.
- Resistance training on machines is usually preferred over free weights because machines require less skill and can be more easily controlled.
- Discontinue any exercise that causes pain or discomfort, and use an alternative exercise. Consult a doctor if you experience any of these warning signs or complications:
1. Vaginal bleeding
2. Abdominal pain or cramping
3. Ruptured membranes
4. Elevated blood pressure or heart rate
5. Lack of foetal movement

reduce intensity if you experience a pounding heart rate, breathlessness or dizziness.
- Eat a small snack before exercising to help avoid hypoglycaemia (low blood sugar).
- Drink plenty of water before, during and after exercise.
- Avoid overstretching or going beyond the normal range of motion.
- Report unusual physical changes (e.g. vaginal bleeding, severe fatigue, joint pain, irregular heartbeat) to your doctor immediately.

It may be a good idea to make contact with a personal trainer in your area who deals specifically with training during pregnancy. You will benefit enormously from working with someone who can offer you an individualized programme.

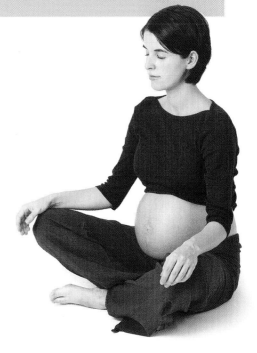

Right: With the number of different changes that are taking place in your body during your pregnancy, it is extremely important to make sure that you always exercise with both caution and awareness.

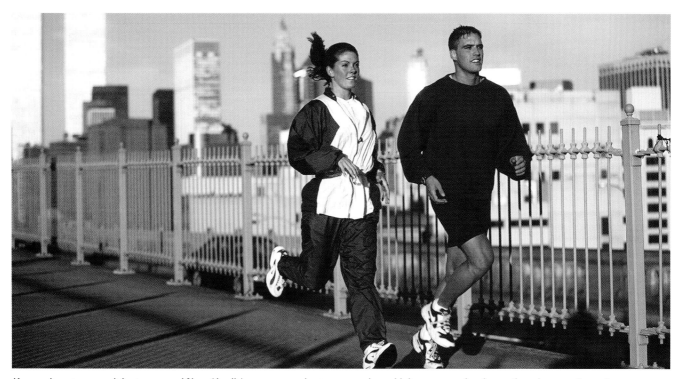

If your long-term goal is to run a 10km (6-mile) race, your short-term goal would be to start jogging a few times each week.

How do you initiate your action plan?

By now you have completed your self-assessments and, together with the information above, you have a good understanding of the components that can make up a physical activity programme. What now?

First, establish why you want to become physically active – something that is covered to some degree in the lifestyle/behaviour assessment on pages 18–19. Do not do it for a nagging partner, doctor, parent or child as you are sure to encounter motivation failure somewhere along the way. Your goals should be yours alone: if you are the one to set them, you will buy in to them more successfully and you will be fully accountable for achieving them.

Long-term goals

This is anything you feel is realistically achievable, usually an event or something similar that excites you to think about completing; examples are running a 10km (6-mile) race, cycling across Africa or losing 5kg (11lb). Setting long-term goals within a four- to 12-month period should work well; anything longer may make it hard to maintain motivation or commitment to your programme; anything shorter and you are moving into dangerous territory, as drop-out tends to occur within the first three months of starting a new programme.

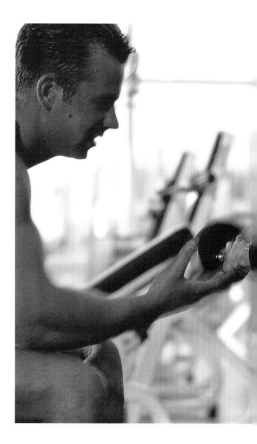

Right: Work with a partner or personal trainer if it will help you stay committed to your programme.

Medium-term goals

These are what help you achieve your long-term goals. For example, if your long-term goal is to lose 8kg (17$^{1}/_{2}$ lb) within four months, your medium-term goal may be to lose 2kg (4$^{1}/_{2}$ lb) per month; if your long-term goal is to run a 10km (6-mile) race within six months, your medium-term goal may be to run 3km (2 miles) by the end of your first month, 5km (3 miles) by the end of your third month, 7.5km (4$^{1}/_{2}$ miles) by the end of your fifth month, etc.

Right: Establish what kind of exercises you enjoy, and include these in your programme to boost your motivation.

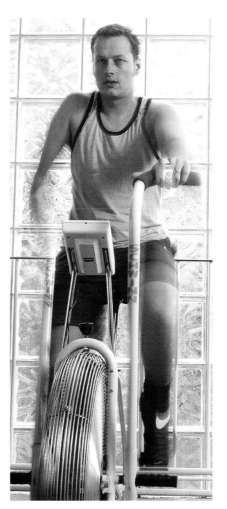

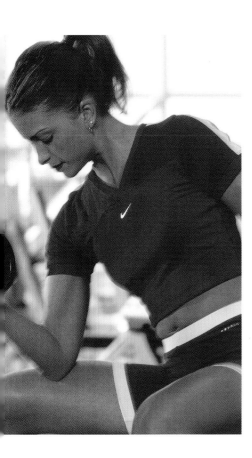

Short-term goals

These are immediate events that facilitate your medium-term goals and may include things as simple as attempting to get to the gym three times a week, stretching for 10 minutes daily or walking during your lunch hour. Make sure these goals are realistic: if you do not normally take a lunch hour, do not opt for a one-hour walk at that time, rather attempt a 10-minute power walk until you become used to the idea of taking time for yourself during your working day.

Together, these short-, medium- and long-term goals make up your *action plan*. Write this plan down so that you can check on it and remind yourself of your goals regularly. Stick it up on your mirror, hang it in the bathroom or attach it somewhere in your car. If you find you hit a rough spot and do not manage to complete your short-term goals for the week, do not panic; simply start up again as soon as you can. If your lapses are happening frequently, you may need to revisit your short- and medium-term goals, perhaps even your long-term goals, as they may not be as realistic as you thought they were. If, however, you are determined to keep the goals you set originally, you may want to consider employing the help of a personal trainer to help you achieve them.

Last, but not least, remember to *reward yourself* when you do achieve your goals consistently, perhaps not with Death by Chocolate double-cream espresso cake, but with a new item of clothing, a weekend away, time by yourself – whatever makes you feel good. You deserve it.

In brief

- Set long-, medium- and short-term goals.
- Write them down and check on them regularly.
- Do not panic if you lapse once or twice; however, revisit and change your goals if you lapse regularly.
- Reward yourself as you achieve your goals.

the Exercise menu

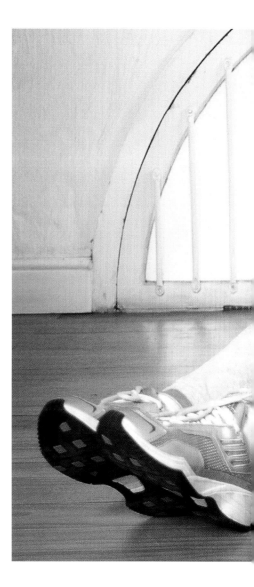

Once you have read Chapter Three to ensure that you understand the principles on which to base your programme, you can start to put everything together by choosing your exercises from the menu provided in this chapter. It has been divided into sections covering *stabilization, resistance training* and *flexibility training*. Since choosing cardio-vascular exercises is based so much on personal taste and enjoyment, the choice of what to include in your programme has been left up to you (*see* page 46β).

Specific guidelines on repetitions have been given in the torso stabilization section since you will not necessarily feel fully fatigued on completion of these exercises, unlike many of the exercises covered under resistance training. The purpose here is to initiate both awareness and activation of stabilization muscles, so a few repetitions performed with good concentration should suffice. Suggestions for repetitions have not been included for either the resistance training or flexibility sections. Refer once again to Chapter Three, where these are covered in some detail (*see* pages 36 and 41). As a guideline for these two types of training methods, remember the following:

- for muscle endurance training: up to 18 or 20 repetitions at a weight that starts to fatigue you at 14 or 15
- to build strength or develop muscle size: up to 10 or 12 repetitions at a weight that starts to fatigue you at seven or eight
- hold stretches for between 30 and 90 seconds.

There are hundreds of resistance and flexibility training exercises, and this book lists only a specific selection for each body part. The selection is based on two premises. The first is that the exercise chosen should be effective in targeting the main muscles responsible for execution of movement. The second is that the exercise can be adapted or simulated to offer the most variety, given that not everyone has access to gym equipment.

This should not, however, stop you from asking a trainer to show you other options to add to your repertoire. Doing the same exercises over and over again can become tedious, so seek alternatives to eliminate boredom. To this end, alternative equipment-based exercises you might prefer to do for each body part are listed in the resistance training section for those who do have access to a gym.

With all the exercises, be sure to keep your deep abdominal muscles activated by pulling your navel to your spine and performing the exercises with focus and control. The actions of contraction and release with resistance – called concentric and eccentric in scientific terms – are equally important and should happen at the same speed and with the same degree of concentration. The more slowly you perform the exercise, the better, as this will eliminate any chance of momentum playing a role in helping you move the weight. Between three and five seconds each for contraction and release should do. Make sure you breathe evenly during your resistance-training workout; avoid holding your breath with exertion, which may cause an increase in your blood pressure.

Some people suggest that exercises in a standing position should be performed with slightly bent knees. The intention is to protect the back, since bending the knees tends to tilt the pelvis forward and put the back into a stretch – eliminating potential compression on the lower back. Functionally, however, it would be better to straighten the legs, without locking the knees, and concentrate on directly activating and strengthening the abdominal muscles so they can offer the back sufficient support. In a sense, you will be forcing them to take responsibility for an optimal pelvic position. Developing pelvic stabilizers will also support you in daily tasks, such as lifting children, picking up shopping, carrying heavy loads of washing, pushing lawnmowers, and so on.

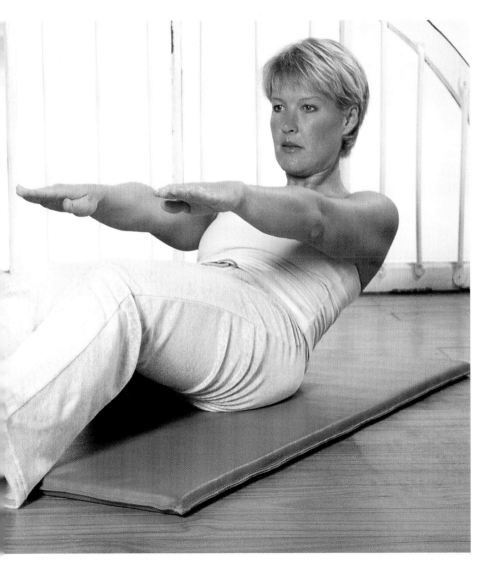

Left: Gym membership is not essential; many exercises can be done without equipment.

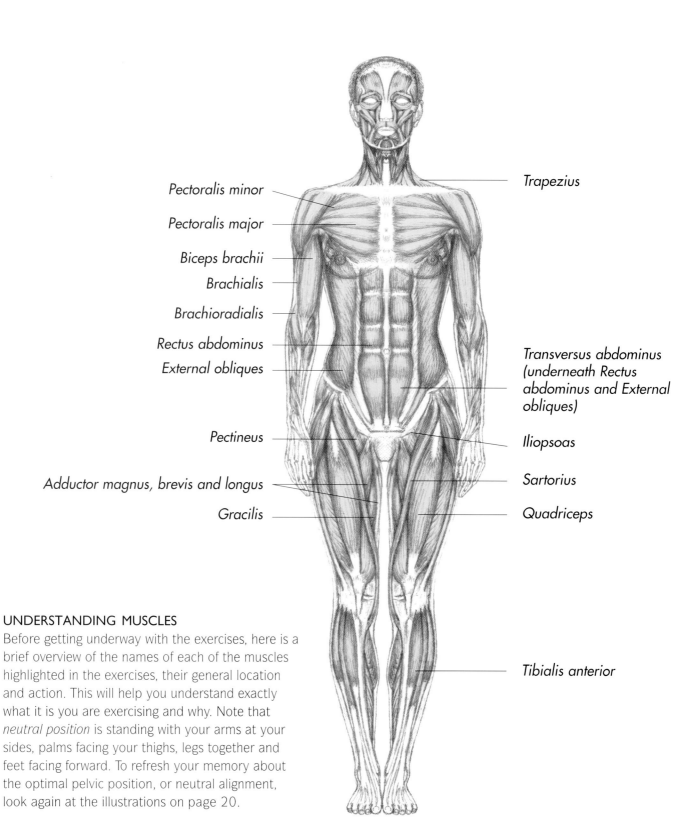

Pectoralis minor

Pectoralis major

Biceps brachii

Brachialis

Brachioradialis

Rectus abdominus

External obliques

Pectineus

Adductor magnus, brevis and longus

Gracilis

Trapezius

Transversus abdominus
(underneath Rectus
abdominus and External
obliques)

Iliopsoas

Sartorius

Quadriceps

Tibialis anterior

UNDERSTANDING MUSCLES

Before getting underway with the exercises, here is a
brief overview of the names of each of the muscles
highlighted in the exercises, their general location
and action. This will help you understand exactly
what it is you are exercising and why. Note that
neutral position is standing with your arms at your
sides, palms facing your thighs, legs together and
feet facing forward. To refresh your memory about
the optimal pelvic position, or neutral alignment,
look again at the illustrations on page 20.

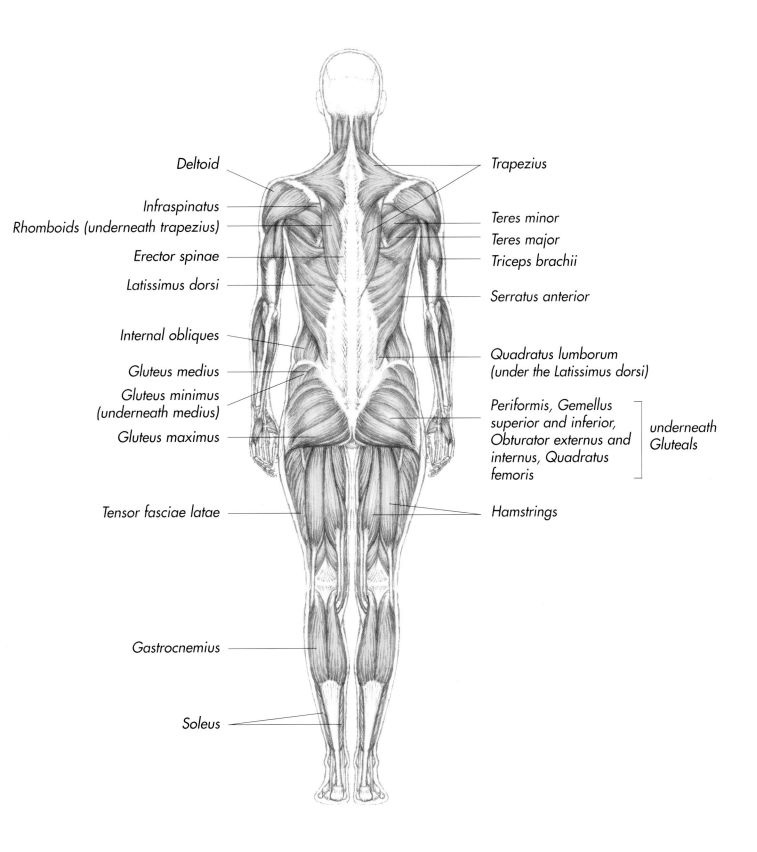

Deltoid

Infraspinatus

Rhomboids (underneath trapezius)

Erector spinae

Latissimus dorsi

Internal obliques

Gluteus medius

Gluteus minimus
(underneath medius)

Gluteus maximus

Tensor fasciae latae

Gastrocnemius

Soleus

Trapezius

Teres minor

Teres major

Triceps brachii

Serratus anterior

Quadratus lumborum
(under the Latissimus dorsi)

Periformis, Gemellus
superior and inferior,
Obturator externus and
internus, Quadratus
femoris

underneath
Gluteals

Hamstrings

Pectorals (chest)

Muscle: *Pectoralis major*
Location: Chest
Action: Internally (inwardly) rotates the arm; moves the arm to the front of the body from a neutral position and draws the arms toward the body

Muscle: *Pectoralis minor*
Location: Top of the chest
Action: Draws the shoulder blades away from one another and assists in depressing them (pulling them down)

Shoulders

Muscle: *Deltoid*
Location: Shoulder
Action: Lifts the arms sideways, forwards and backwards away from the body and rotates them both internally (inwardly) as well as externally (outwardly)

Arms

Muscle: *Triceps brachii*
Location: Back of the upper arm
Action: Straightens the elbow and moves the arm backwards away from the body through the neutral position

Muscle: *Biceps brachii*
Location: Front of the upper arm
Action: Bends the elbow; internally rotates the forearm and helps to move the arm upwards towards the front of the body

Muscle: *Brachioradialis*
Location: Forearm
Action: Bends the elbow and internally and externally rotates the forearm

Muscle: *Brachialis*
Location: Forearm
Action: Bends the elbow

Back

Muscle: *Trapezius*
Location: Upper, middle and lower back, close to the spine
Action: Lifts, depresses and pulls the shoulder blades together

Muscle: *Quadratus lumborum*
Location: Lower back
Action: Bends the spine to the side and stabilizes the pelvis and lower (lumbar) spine

Muscle: *Serratus anterior*
Location: Surface of the ribs
Action: Pulls the shoulder blades away from the spine and flatten them against the back

Muscle: *Rhomboids*
Location: Between shoulder blades
Action: Pulls shoulder blades together

Muscle: *Latissimus dorsi*
Location: Lower and middle back
Action: Draws the arms toward the body, moves them from in front of the body to behind the body through the neutral position, and internally rotates them

Muscle: *Teres major*
Location: Back of the shoulder blade
Action: Moves the arms backwards through the neutral position, internally rotates them and draws them toward one another

Muscle: *Erector spinae*
Location: Long muscles running along the length of the spine
Action: Extends and bends the spine sideways

Muscle: *Infraspinatus*
Location: Back of the shoulder blade
Action: Externally rotates the arms and lifts them backwards from the neutral position

Muscle: *Teres minor*
Location: Back of the shoulder joint
Action: As above

Abdominals

Muscle: *Transversus abdominus*
Location: Deep into the abdominal region
Action: Stabilizes the pelvis

Muscle: *Internal, external obliques*
Location: Waist
Action: Rotates the lower spine and bends it sideways and forwards

Muscle: *Rectus abdominus*
Location: Front of ribs and pelvis
Action: Bends the spine to the side and bends the lower spine forwards

Hips

Muscle: *Pectineus*
Location: Front of the pubis
Action: Bends the hip joint, internally rotates the legs and draws them toward the neutral position

Muscle: *Iliopsoas*
Location: Front of pelvis
Action: Bends the hip joint and externally rotates the legs

Legs

Muscle: *Hamstrings*
Location: Back of leg
Action: Bends the knee, externally and internally rotates the leg and knee, and extends the hip joint

Muscle: *Quadriceps*
Location: Front of thigh
Action: Bends the hip joint as well as straightens the knee

Muscle: *Tensor fasciae latae*
Location: Outside of the leg
Action: Pulls the legs sideways away from the neutral position, bends the hip joints and rotates the legs internally at the same time

Muscle: *Adductor magnus, brevis and longus*
Location: Inner thigh
Action: Draws the legs inward toward the neutral position, externally rotates them and assists in bending the hip joint

Muscle: *Gracilis*
Location: Inner thigh
Action: Draws the legs inward toward the neutral position, bends the knees and internally rotates the legs

Buttocks
Muscle: *Gluteus medius*
Location: Side of buttocks
Action: Pulls the legs sideways away from the neutral position and both externally and internally rotates them

Muscle: *Gluteus maximus*
Location: Buttocks
Action: Extends the hip as well as externally rotates the legs

Muscle: *Gluteus minimus*
Location: Side of buttocks
Action: Pulls the legs sideways away from the neutral position and internally rotates them as it does so

Muscles: *Periformis, gemellus superior and inferior, obturator externus and internus, quadratus femoris*
Location: Buttocks
Action: External rotation of the hip (leg)

Calves
Muscle: *Gastrocnemius*
Location: Calf
Action: Points the feet and bends the knees

Muscle: *Soleus*
Location: Calf
Action: Points the feet

Muscle: *Tibialis anterior*
Location: Shin
Action: Flexes the feet, pulling the toes toward the shin, and inverts or rolls the feet outward

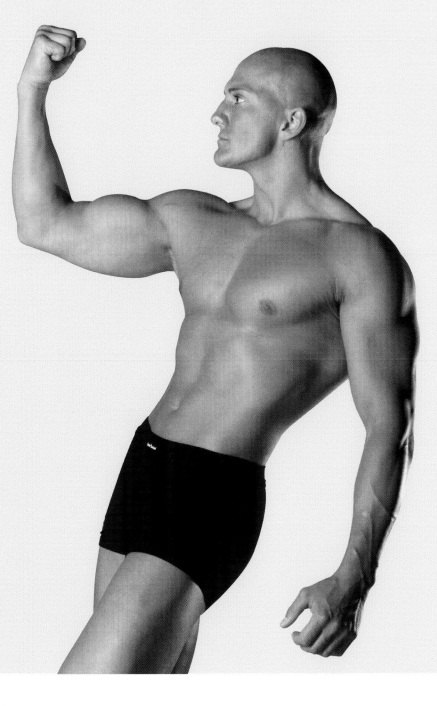

Torso stabilization

Upright standing pose

This is an excellent position to work from when standing to perform exercises. Use it as often as possible throughout your day to activate the main postural stabilizers.

Why: Creates postural awareness.

How

Feet: Balance your weight on your feet – front and back, inner and outer, and on the right and left foot. Keep your heels pressed down as you (mentally) lift your ankles and shin bones.

Legs: Pull up your front thigh muscles and rotate your inner thighs circularly inward (in an anti-clockwise direction on the right leg and a clockwise direction on the left – the reverse of the classic 'turned-out' ballet stance). Remain conscious of your outer thighs rotating at the same time. This will help to open up the lower back by creating space in that area. Rotating the legs in the opposite direction tends to compress the lower back.

Trunk: Lengthen your waist and lift your chest bone without sticking your ribs out. Keep your shoulders back, with your shoulder blades flattened into your back. Maintain a neutral pelvic position. Keep shoulders and arms relaxed.

Neck: Lengthen your neck and balance your head above your legs, with your chin parallel to the floor; do not tuck it down or tilt it up.

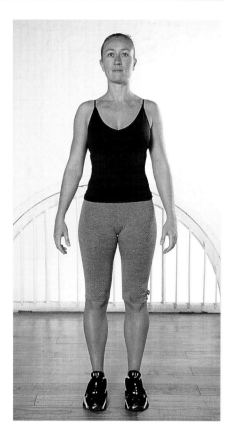

Seated ball balance

Why: Improves awareness and strength of posture.

How

Beginners: Sit on a stability ball, with your hands off the ball at your sides, feet on the ground and ankles placed directly underneath your knees. Activate your abdominal stabilizers by pulling your navel to your spine and ensuring that your pelvis is in a neutral position.

Intermediate/advanced: As above, but slowly lift one knee upward about 15cm (6in) off the floor. Ensuring that your spine remains in its neutral position, without tilting sideways, backwards or forwards, and that your hips and shoulders remain facing to the front, hold the knee where it is for a couple of seconds before lowering and repeating on the other side. Keep your chin parallel to the floor.

Repetitions: 5–6 on each side

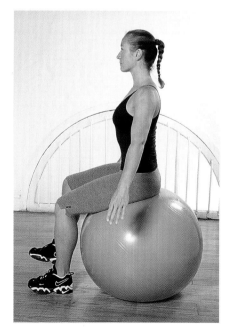

Back roll

Why: This exercise increases mobility of the spine. Many people appear to have fairly immobile lower backs; when asked to stand and roll their torsos forward and downward towards the floor, they bend from the hips instead of from the spine. This may be as a result of tight back muscles, injury, or intervertebral disc problems, etc. Whatever the cause, it may result in the spine becoming less mobile.

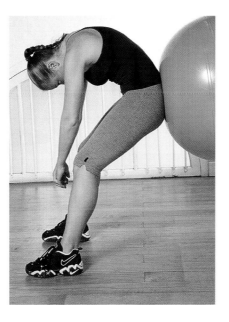 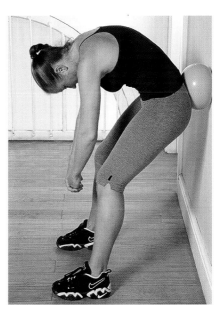

How

Stand against a wall with a ball placed against the bottom of your lower back. Your feet should be planted fairly wide and forward of the body in a semi-squat position. Starting by tucking your chin in, slowly roll your head, neck and spine downward towards the feet until your hands almost touch the floor, ensuring that you keep your lower back against the ball for as long as possible. Watch out for any flattening of your lower back and try not to let your legs bend any further than when you began the exercise. Roll back upward in a similar way. Your navel should be pulled towards the spine at all times during this exercise.

Repetitions: 5–6

Alternative: Do the exercise using a small play ball.

Forward ball roll

Why: Strengthens the abdominals, back, pelvis and shoulder area.

How

Intermediate/advanced: Kneel with legs slightly apart in front of a stability ball, with your forearms placed on the ball. Pull your navel toward your spine, depress your shoulders and ensure that your pelvis is in neutral alignment. Slowly roll the ball forward, keeping the correct pelvic position. Return to the starting position and repeat, ensuring throughout the exercise that you do not allow your lower back to arch.

Repetitions: 5–6

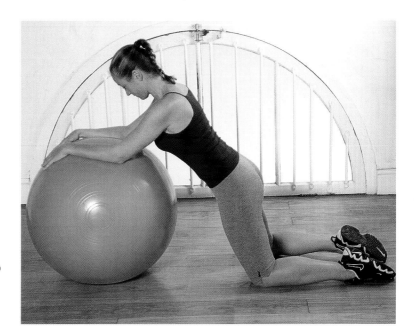

Hitcher

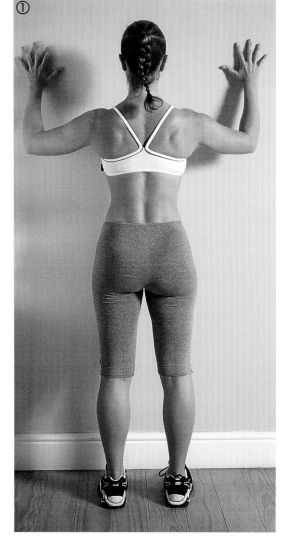

Why: Strengthens middle and lower trapezius muscle. The trapezius is kite-shaped (*see* pages 56–57), and the uppermost and smallest part of it tends to work harder than the lower, largest part. Habitually incorrect posture and seated deskwork often lead to this imbalance, with the upper back taking most of the tension. General stiffness and discomfort, as well as tension headaches, can stem from a tight neck and back of the shoulder area. At the same time, the middle and lower back are put into a stretch due to slouching, which tends to weaken these muscles over time.

How

① **Beginners:** Stand facing a wall, with elbows bent at right angles just below shoulder height and palms lightly touching the wall. Pull your navel towards your spine and slowly draw your shoulder blades down towards your buttocks, being careful not to drop your elbows. Hold for one to four slow counts and then release.

② **Intermediate:** Lie face down on a narrow gym bench or a corner of a bed or table, with your arms hanging down toward the floor. Slowly raise your arms forward and outward until the elbows are bent at right angles just below shoulder level. Your palms should be facing your head, with your thumbs pointing upwards to the ceiling – hence the name 'hitcher'. Keep your shoulders and neck completely relaxed. In this position, draw your shoulder blades down toward your buttocks. Hold for one to four slow counts and then release the arms back to the floor.
Repetitions: 10–12

③ **Advanced:** As for previous exercise, but perform the exercise on a stability ball, with the feet resting on the floor.

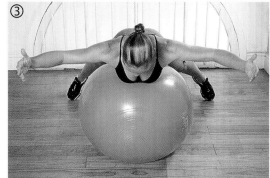

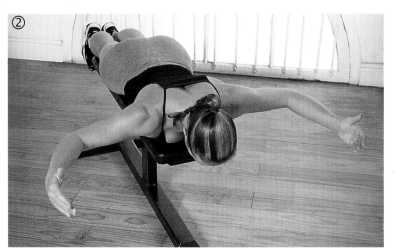

Reading pose

Why: Strengthens the serratus anterior. It is important to strengthen this muscle if your shoulders are hunched or roll forward. People with this problem often also have tight chests so this exercise, coupled with a good chest stretch (*see* pages 89–90), can do wonders for improving posture.

How

Beginners: Lie face down on the floor, supporting yourself on your elbows, which should be placed directly underneath your shoulders. Put your palms flat against the floor. Depress your shoulders and activate your abdominal muscles by pulling your navel to your spine, so that your abdomen is raised off the floor and your back is lengthened. This pose looks similar to that of someone lying reading a book.

Intermediate/advanced: This exercise can be performed on the hands, with straight arms, feet on floor, legs straight and knees off the floor (*intermediate*, see picture ② on page 64); or on the elbows, with feet on the floor, legs straight and knees off the floor (*advanced*, see picture ③ on page 64).

Repetitions: Hold for as long as you can keep your shoulders down and abdomen lifted – about a minute. It is harder than it looks.

✍ Trainer's tip

Try to avoid squeezing your buttocks as this diminishes the space in your lower back, which you need in order to achieve good lengthening of the spine.

Alternative: An easier version is with wider elbows, so that you are working closer to the ground.

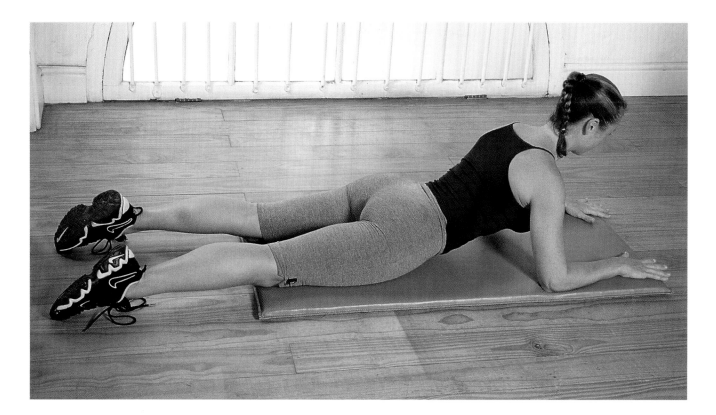

Abdominal plank pose

Why: Strengthens the abdominal muscles. The abdominals, particularly the transversus abdominus, which is the deepest abdominal muscle, are some of the most important muscles involved in trunk stability. They are therefore vital for ensuring neutral alignment of the spine. Strengthening these muscles can often diminish general back pain associated with excessive lower-back arching or compression.

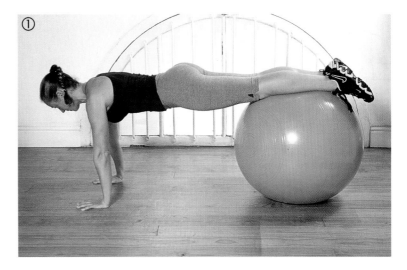

How

① Lie face down on a stability ball and slowly roll your body forward so that eventually either your thighs (*beginners*), top of shins (*intermediate*) or feet (*advanced*) are the only body parts left on the ball. With your hands on the floor and placed directly underneath the shoulders, hold this position with your navel pulled to your spine and your shoulders depressed and flattened against your back.

Repetitions: Hold for about 30 seconds or as long as you are able to keep neutral alignment of the spine.

Alternative: This exercise can also be performed on the hands, with the feet on the floor, legs straight and knees off the floor (*intermediate* ②), or on the elbows, with the feet on the floor, legs straight and knees off the floor (*advanced* ③).

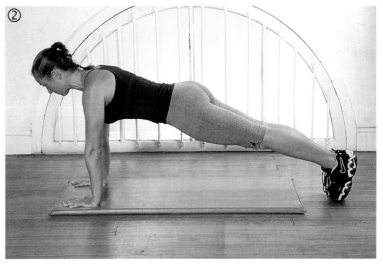

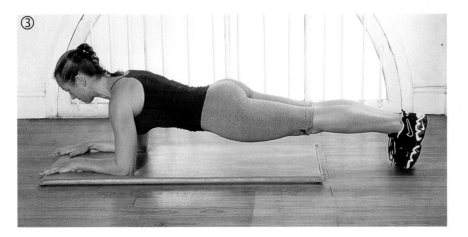

✐ Trainer's tip

Do not allow your lower back to sag. You should not experience back pain in this exercise; if you do, it is possible that you are either working too far off the ball, or you are not activating the abdominals effectively.

Transverse activator

Why: Strengthens the deepest abdominal muscle.

How

① Kneel sideways to a mirror on all fours, with your hands under your shoulders and your knees under your hips. Keep your spine in a neutral curvature (that is, with a very slight lower-back arch) and take a deep breath in. Slowly breathe out, while pulling your navel to your spine, so that you actually see your abdominals moving upwards. Do not change the relaxed position of your spine while performing the exercise.

Repetitions: 10–12

② **Alternative:** Lie face down on the floor with your arms under your forehead. Relax your back completely and take a deep breath in. Slowly breathe out while pulling your navel to your spine, so that a space is created between the floor and your stomach. Again, do not change the position of your spine while performing the exercise.

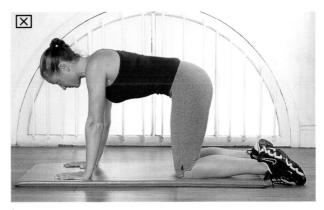

Incorrect

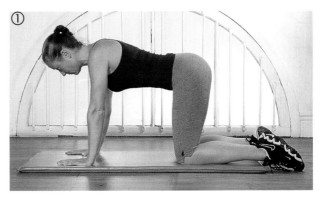

Correct

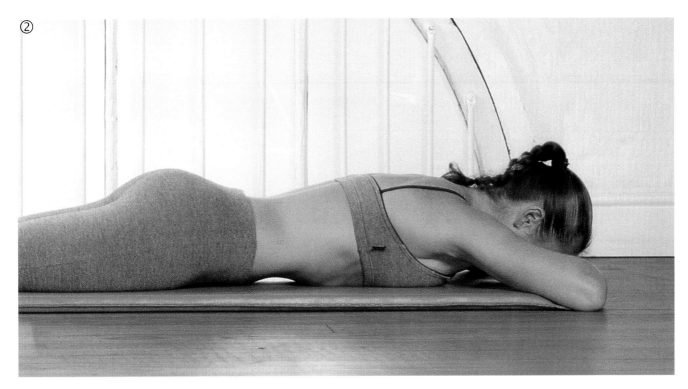

Leaning side support

Why: Strengthens the internal and external obliques and quadratus lumborum.

How

① **Beginners:** Sit on your right hip with the knees bent and in line with, or slightly forward of the hips. Leaning on either the elbow (easier) or hand (harder) of the right arm, slowly raise your hips sideways off the floor. Try to imagine you are lying sideways on a board, so that your knees, hips and shoulders are in line with one another. Keeping your shoulders relaxed and your navel pulled to your spine, hold for about five seconds or longer if you can before lowering back to the floor. Repeat on the left side.

② **Intermediate:** As above, but use a straight supporting arm.

③ **Advanced:** As above but straighten your legs in the starting position. Ensure that your feet are in line with your hips, not behind.

Repetitions: 2 to each side

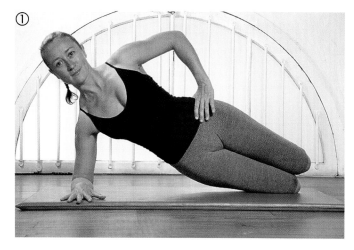

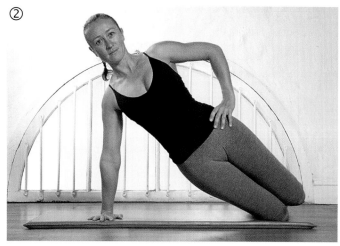

Resistance training

Pectorals (chest)

Push-ups

Type: Compound exercise
Main muscle: Pectoralis major
Other muscles: Deltoids, pectoralis minor, serratus anterior, triceps

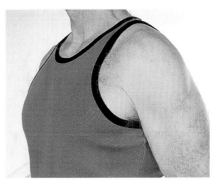

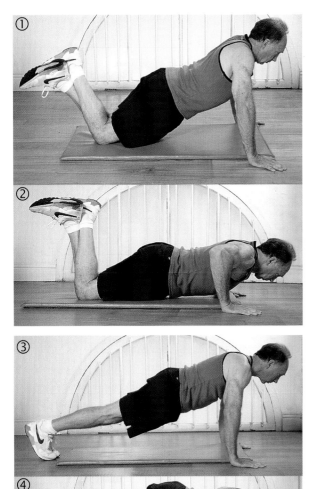

How

①–② **Beginners:** Kneel on the floor with your feet crossed, knees together and hands on the floor, slightly forward of and wider than your shoulders. Ensure that your knees, hips and shoulders are in a diagonal line. Slowly lower your body to the floor in this same position and then push up to start again. If you cannot manage a full push-up, take it halfway down until your strength improves.

③–④ **Intermediate/advanced:** As above, but on your feet rather than on the knees, keeping your legs straight. Keeping your body completely straight, slowly lower yourself to the floor, aiming to touch the floor with your chest and pubic bone.

⑤ **Very advanced:** Perform your push-up with your feet up on a raised object, such as a step or a stability ball.

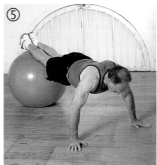

✎ Trainer's tip

To avoid arching in the lower back, keep your navel pulled hard in toward your spine and try to imagine the effort or exertion coming from your chest.

Flyes

Type: Isolation exercise
Main muscle: Pectoralis major

✍ Trainer's tip

Many people do this exercise

without arm rotation. Since one of

the functions of the pectoralis major

is to internally rotate the arm, it

makes sense to bring in the rotation

factor while exercising this muscle.

How

①–② **Beginners:** Lie on your back on the floor or a bench, with your feet placed in front of your buttocks, knees bent. With your selected weight in your hands, start with the arms straight and directly above the chest (in line with your nipples), with the backs of the hands facing each other. Although your arms should be straight, do not lock your elbows but keep them slightly soft.

Slowly open out the hands toward the floor, turning the palms to face the ceiling as you go and stopping when the hands line up horizontally with the shoulders. If on a bench, do not drop the arms any further down than the level of the bench, as it may overstretch and place unnecessary load on the shoulder joints.
Return to the starting position.

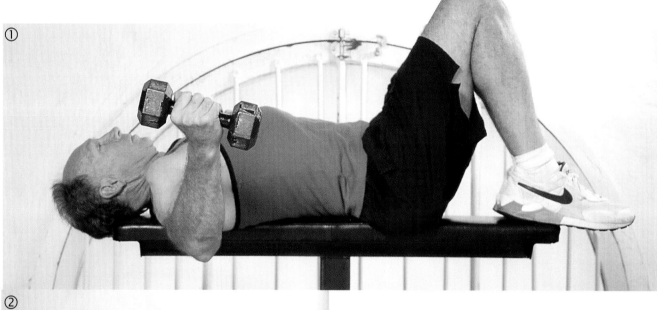

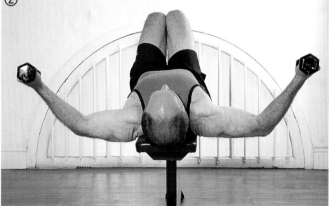

③ **Alternative:** Lie on the floor and place a stretch band underneath your upper back, holding on to each end with your hands. Perform the exercise as above.

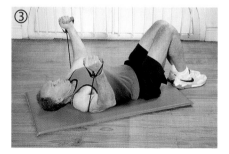

Cable cross-over

Type: Compound exercise
Main muscle: Pectoralis major
Other muscles: Deltoids, abdominals

How

① This exercise can be done using either the upper or lower cables of a cable cross-over – if you have access to one in your gym – to target the upper or lower fibres of the chest, respectively. Stand between and with the cables in each hand, palms facing down. Place one foot forward of the other for stability and bend both knees slightly. Leaning forward in the chest to a 45-degree angle, slowly bring the hands downwards and forwards, so that they end up in front of your chest, in line with your nipples, with the backs of the hands almost touching. Release back to starting position again.

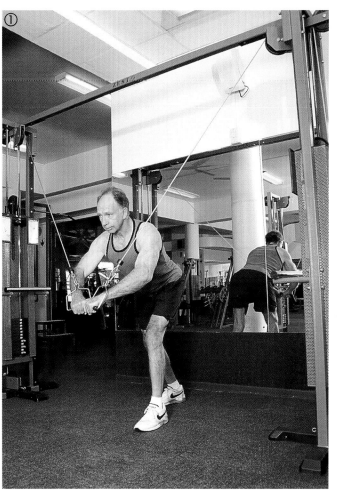

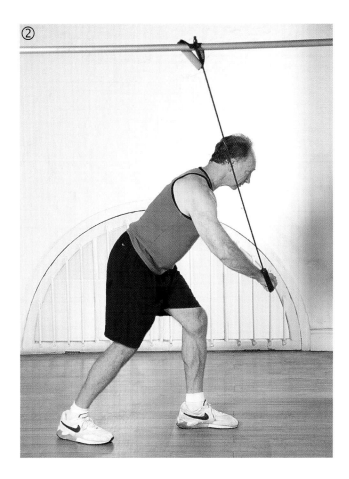

② **Alternative:** Attach a stretch band to a shower or curtain rail and do the exercise, one side at a time, ensuring that you continue to maintain good posture and a motionless torso.

✎ Trainer's tip

As for the flyes exercise opposite (see page 68).

Further exercises

Lying bench press (incline, decline, flat); seated chest press; pec deck

Deltoids (shoulder muscles)

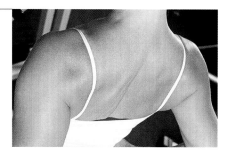

Narrow arm push-ups

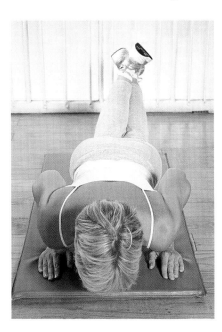

Type: Compound exercise
Main muscles: Anterior deltoid and triceps
Other muscles: Pectorals

How

As with the regular push-up exercise (*see* page 67), but keep your hands directly underneath and no wider than your shoulders, with the fingers facing directly forward. Slowly lower yourself to the floor, keeping your elbows tucked into your sides, so that they brush your waist on the way down.

✎ *Trainer's tip*

Avoid 'winging' your elbows out to the sides, since this will detract from the tricep action.

Side raises

Type: Isolation exercise
Main muscle: Middle deltoid

How

① Using the 'upright standing pose' explained on page 60, stand with your hands at your sides and palms facing your legs. With your selected weight slowly lift your arms to the side, turning your palms outward, so that your palms face the front at the top of the movement. Take hands to chin height but no higher, as this could overwork and strain the neck. Slowly lower the arms back to the starting position.
② **Alternative:** Hook a stretch band under your feet and clasp the ends in your hands. Do as above.

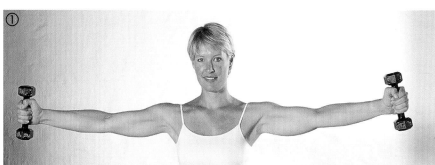

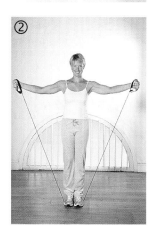

✎ *Trainer's tip*

Use the muscle activated in the 'hitcher' exercise (see page 62). By maintaining trunk stability, this helps to isolate the shoulder muscles and make this exercise effective. The rotation action allows more freedom in the shoulder joint.

Front raises

Type: Isolation exercise
Main muscle: Anterior deltoid

How

① As with the previous exercise, but this time lift your arms diagonally to the front (not directly to the front) of your body. When raising the hands, keep the palms facing the floor.
② **Alternative:** Hook a stretch band under your feet and clasp the ends in your hands. Do as above.

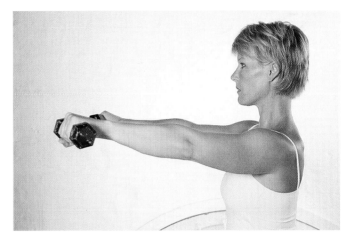

✍ Trainer's tip

Try to employ the muscle activated in the 'hitcher' exercise (see page 62). At the angle used in this exercise, there is less of an issue with tightness in the shoulder joint than in the 'side raises' opposite, so internal rotation, which is one of the functions of the front deltoid, can be used.

Back raises

Type: Compound exercise
Main muscle: Posterior deltoid
Other muscles: Triceps

How

① Stand with both knees bent and feet slightly apart, with your arms at your side and palms facing your thighs. Tilt your chest slightly forward to approximately 30 degrees. Slowly raise your arms to the back, while turning your palms outward, away from your body. Raise your arms as far as you can without changing the position of your body.
② **Alternative:** Hook a stretch band around your feet and clasp the ends in your hand. Do as above.

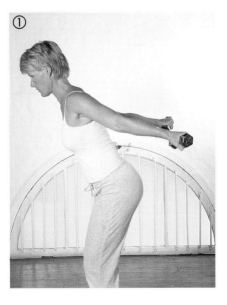

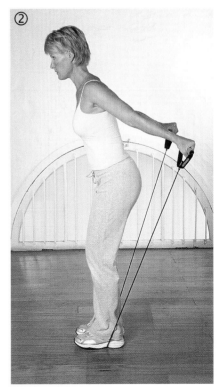

Further exercises

Shoulder press (decline, upright)

✍ Trainer's tip

Avoid tilting your body further in order to get your arms higher.

Arms

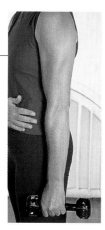

External arm rotators

The external rotators of the arms are often fairly weak, as most of the movements we perform daily tend to use the muscles that rotate the arms inward. As most of the exercises provided here also strengthen the internal rotators, adding this one to your programme will protect against possible arm muscle imbalances.

Type: Compound exercise

Main muscles: Infraspinatus, teres minor

How

① Lie on one side, with your knees bent and feet forward of your hips. Lay your head down onto the arm closest to the floor, which should be extended above your head. With your chosen weight in your free hand and with your elbow bent and tucked into your waist, slowly lift the weight upward toward the ceiling, keeping your shoulders and hips facing the front. Once you have gone as high as you can without displacing your shoulders or hips, slowly lower your hand to the floor. Your hand should remain in line with your elbow throughout this exercise. Repeat on the other side.

②–③ **Alternative:** This exercise can be performed standing, with a stretch band tied around a door handle. With the band held in the hand furthest away from the handle and with your body turned so that the band stretches across the front of your body, slowly pull the band as far away from the handle as possible, ensuring that your hips and shoulders remain facing the front. The hand of the working arm should be in line with the elbow, which is tucked into your waist.

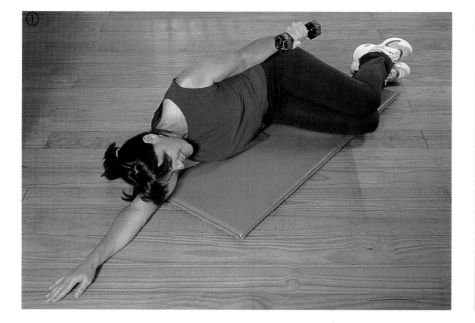

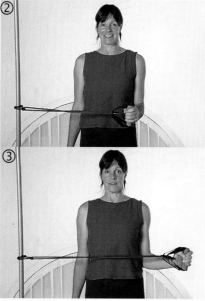

Dips

Type: Compound exercise
Main muscle: Triceps
Other muscles: Rhomboids, deltoids, triceps, latissimus dorsi, teres major

How

Use either a seated dip machine or hanging dip bar in your gym, or work off the inside of the corner of a countertop in your home or office. With your elbows straight and your hands placed just wider than shoulder-width apart, keep your shoulders depressed (more than in the picture). Bend your elbows and shift your torso forward about 10 or 15 degrees as you lower your body downwards. Try not to take your shoulders into an angle deeper than 45 degrees, as this puts unnecessary strain and stretch on this fairly vulnerable joint. Push upward again to the starting position, ensuring that your shoulders stay down throughout the exercise.
Beginners: The seated dip machine is your best option. If you do not have access to one, perform the exercises as described above but ask someone to help you by holding your feet and lowering you as your elbows bend, then giving you a thrust back up to your starting point again. As you get stronger, try lowering your body by yourself.

✎ Trainer's tip

The wider your grip in this exercise, the more back muscles you will bring in; the narrower your grip, the more arm and shoulder muscles you will activate.

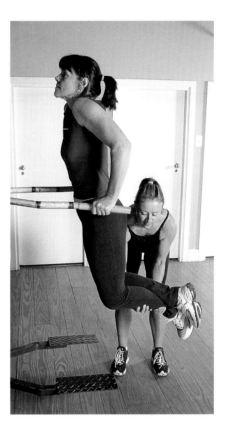

Tricep push-down

Type: Isolation exercise
Main muscle: Triceps

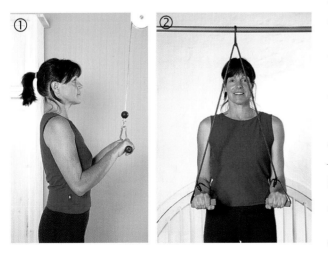

How

① Using the tricep pushdown machine, grip the bar with your hands no wider than shoulder-width apart and slowly bring your arms down until your elbows touch your waist. This is the first stage of the exercise. In the second stage, bring your hands down toward your thighs, keeping the elbows tucked in at your waist. Slowly take the bar back to the starting position again.
② **Alternative:** Tie a stretch band around a shower or curtain rail and clasp the ends in each hand. Do as above.

✎ Trainer's tip

Do not allow your shoulders to lift up or roll forward. Try instead to employ the muscle activated in the 'hitcher' exercise on page 62.

Dual overhead tricep extension / overarm pullover

Type: Compound exercise
Main muscle: Triceps
Other muscles: Latissimus dorsi, teres major

How

①–③ Lie on your back on a bench (or the end of a bed), with your knees bent and feet up close to your buttocks. Select your weight based on the fact that you will be working with one dumbbell, barbell or makeshift weight. Clasp the weight in both hands, palms facing each other and elbows bent at a 90-degree angle. The weight should be above or behind your head, depending on your level of flexibility and strength; the elbows should be placed anywhere from pointing up to the ceiling, to the wall ahead of you. Keeping your navel pulled in towards your spine, slowly extend the arms, ensuring that you keep your elbows at their initial height. Then take the arms forward toward the pubic bone, stopping when they are above your navel. Slowly move back to the start again.

④–⑤ **Alternative:** As this is an awkward exercise to do with a stretch band (your head gets in the way), an alternative overhead tricep extension exercise is to sit with your left hand behind your lower back, palm facing outward and holding one end of the band. With right elbow bent and pointing toward the ceiling (next to your right ear), hold the other end of the band and slowly extend it overhead. Ensure your right shoulder remains depressed and your bent elbow stays facing the ceiling and against your ear. Repeat on other side.

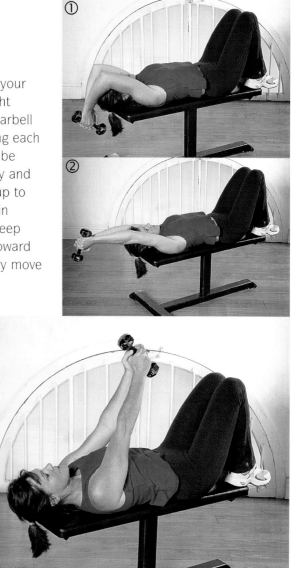

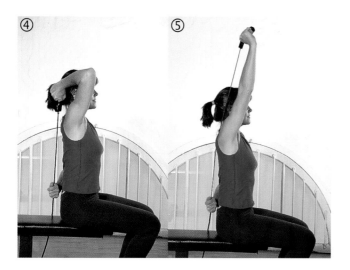

✎ Trainer's tip

To increase the difficulty of this exercise ①–③, squeeze the sides of your head with your elbows and drop the elbows as low as they can go next to your head.

①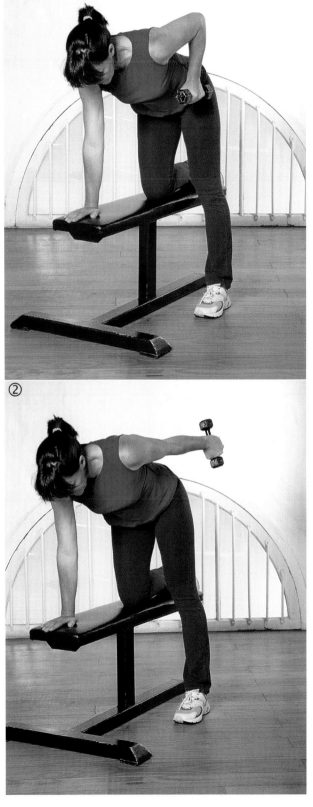

②

Tricep extension

Type: Isolation exercise
Main muscle: Triceps brachii

How

①–② Kneel on one knee on a bench (or similar surface) with the other foot on the floor for stability. Using the same hand as the knee raised, put it on the same surface and forward of that knee, so that your torso is supported while leaning forward. Holding your chosen weight in the opposite hand, bend your elbow upward toward the ceiling, keeping the arm tucked in close to the waist. Slowly extend your hand backwards until your elbow straightens. Lower back down to your starting position again. Repeat on the other side.

③–④ **Alternative:** Wrap a stretch band around the back of your neck, hold the ends in each hand and slowly extend both arms slowly backward, keeping your elbows tucked in to your sides and as far back as is possible with relaxed shoulders.

✎ Trainer's tip

The higher you keep your elbow, the harder this exercise becomes. Always keep the shoulders down.

③ 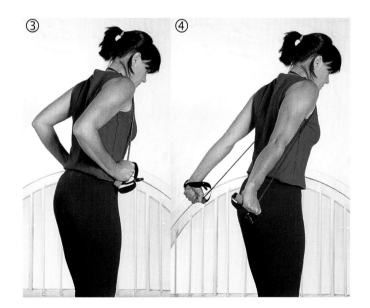 ④

Bicep curl

Type: Compound exercise
Main muscles: Biceps brachii, brachialis, brachioradialis

How

①–② Using the 'upright standing pose' explained on page 60, stand with your selected weights in hand and your palms facing forward. Slowly lift your hands upward toward your shoulders, bending your elbows. Once you touch your shoulders, lower the hands down to the starting position again.
③–④ **Alternative:** The same exercise can be done with a stretch band hooked under the feet.

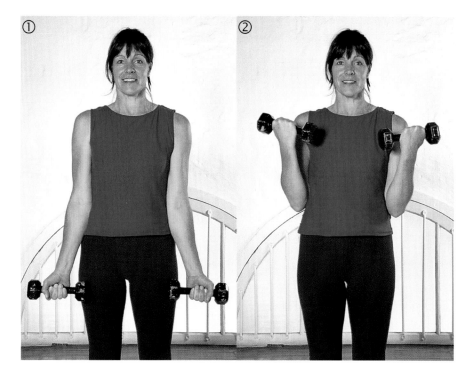

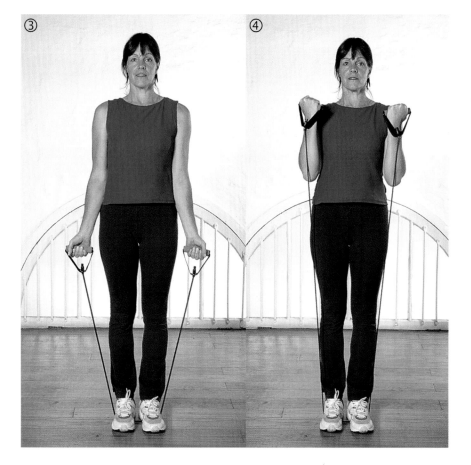

> ✎ *Trainer's tip*
>
> *Keep your body absolutely still to*
>
> *avoid using momentum to help you.*

Further exercises

Seated tricep pushdown

Back

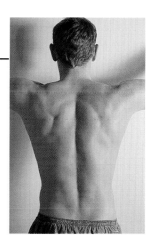

Lying multi-limb extension

Type: Compound exercise
Main muscles: Erector spinae, gluteals, hamstrings
Other muscles: Deltoids, rhomboids

How

① **Intermediate/advanced:** Lie face down on a stability ball with your feet and hands lightly touching the floor. Ensure that you are feeling stable in this position before slowly lifting your left arm to the side. Once you have balance, lift your right leg backwards off the floor. Both arm and leg should end up parallel to the floor – no higher. Hold for about three or four seconds in a stable balance and then repeat on the other side.

② **Alternative:** A more stable version of this exercise for beginners can be done lying face down on the floor, lifting the opposite arm and leg approximately 10 to 20 degrees off the floor.

✎ Trainer's tip

If you want to target your buttocks more on this exercise, externally rotate (turn outward) the leg that you are raising.

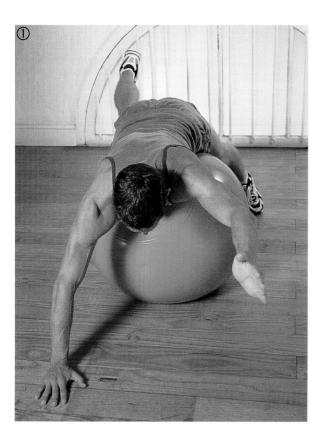

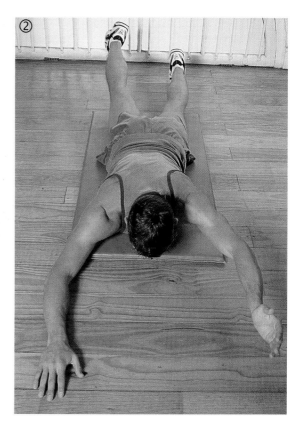

Back extension

This exercise should not be performed by anyone at risk of lower-back injury. If you experience any lower-back pain, use the kneeling single-leg extension opposite instead.

Type: Isolation exercise
Main muscle: Erector spinae

How

① **Beginners:** Lie face down on the floor with your hands next to your thighs. Keep your feet on the floor and legs turned slightly outward. This brings in the buttock muscles to help the back muscles in this exercise. Slowly raise your chest off the floor as high as you can, ensuring that you lengthen the spine as much as possible. Aim for the corner of the ceiling and wall opposite you, rather than the ceiling above you.

② **Intermediate:** As above, but with your hands under your forehead.

③ **Advanced:** As above, but with your hands clasped behind your head. To eliminate the buttock assistance, release this muscle and try to keep your ankles and knees touching.

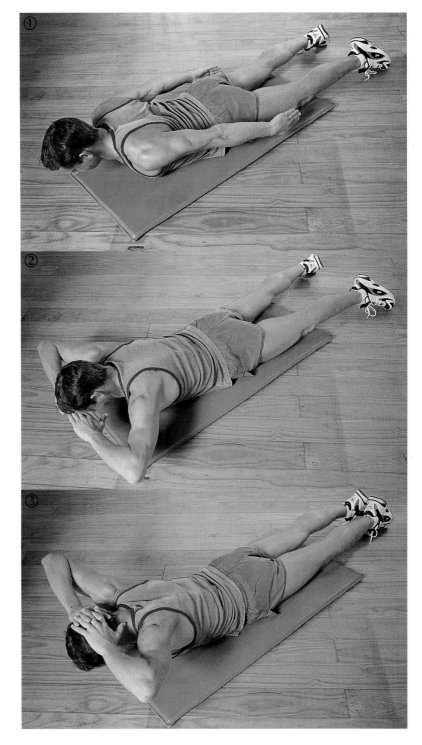

✐ Trainer's tip

Keep your shoulders depressed throughout this exercise and aim to activate the muscle highlighted in the 'hitcher' exercise (see page 62).

Kneeling single-leg extension

Type: Compound exercise
Main muscles: Erector spinae, gluteals, hamstrings
Other muscles: Abdominals

How

① **Beginners:** Kneel on your hands and knees. Keeping your weight even between all four points of contact, slowly lift one leg backwards, straightening the knee until the back of your thigh is in line with your buttocks. Do not twist the hips or shoulders at the top of the movement. Your navel should be pulled to your spine throughout the exercise. Repeat on the other side.

② **Intermediate:** As above, but lift the opposite hand to the knee raised and hold for a few seconds, ensuring that your weight is evenly balanced between both points of contact.

✎ Trainer's tip

The most important thing in this exercise is to avoid arching your lower back, as this can cause compression in this area.

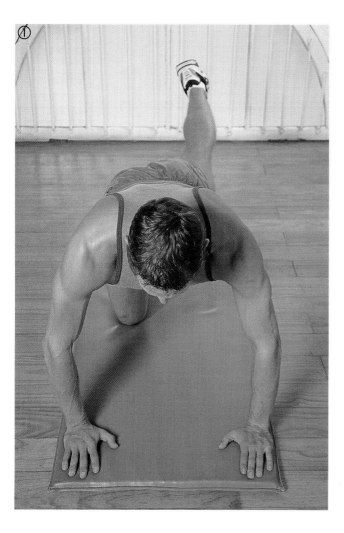

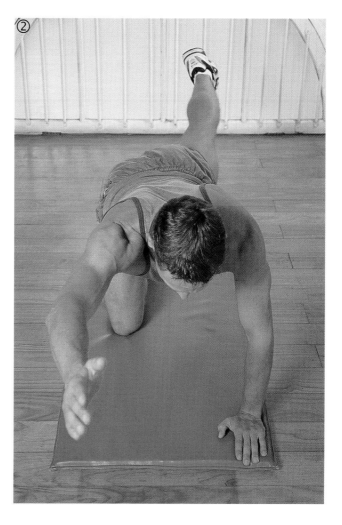

Lat (latissimus) pulldown

Type: Compound exercise
Main muscles: Latissimus dorsi, biceps, brachialis, brachioradialis
Other muscles: Teres major, rhomboids, abdominals, mid-trapezius

🔖 *Trainer's tip*

Although this exercise is called a lat pulldown, when it is performed to the back of the neck it tends to omit one of the three main functions of the latissimus muscles, which is internal rotation of the arm.

How

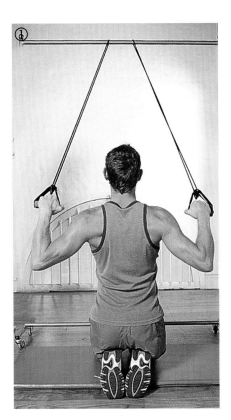

① Sit at a pulldown bar (or with stretch bands tied to a shower or curtain rail), with your hands clasping the bar slightly wider than shoulder-width apart. Lean your torso back about 15 or 20 degrees as you bring the bar downward toward the top of your chest, with the elbows moving backwards as far as possible. Keep your chin tucked in and your shoulders relaxed and your chest open. Ensure that you keep your navel pulled into your spine throughout, so that your lower back does not arch. Hold the bar at the bottom of this exercise for a few seconds and then slowly release it back up again, keeping the elbows tucked in toward the body.

② **Alternative:** Stand with both arms in front of the body at chest height, holding a stretch band, palms facing one another. Slowly lower the right arm toward the side of your body and then continue backwards until it ends up as far behind you as you can go, while maintaining good form. Do not allow the right shoulder to roll forward. Internally rotate the arm as you perform this exercise. Repeat on the other side.

🔖 *Trainer's tip*

You will need to stabilize the non-working arm well in order to retain the arm position. Ensure that you are using your abdominal stabilizers, as well as the muscle groups employed during the 'hitcher' and 'reading' exercises (covered in the earlier Torso Stabilization section, see pages 62 and 63).

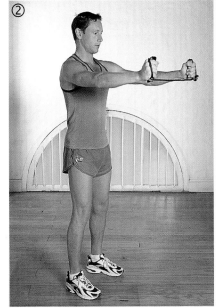

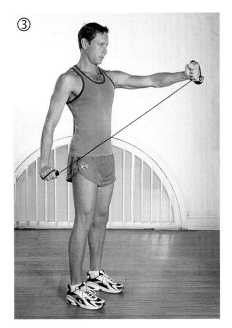

Chin-ups

Type: Compound exercise
Main muscles: Latissimus dorsi, biceps, brachialis, brachioradialis
Other muscles: Teres major, rhomboids, abdominals, posterior deltoid, mid-trapezius

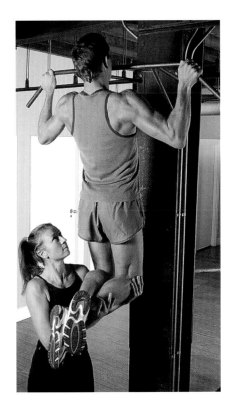

How

Find a bar from which you can hang – either a chin-up bar in a gym, or the top frame of a jungle gym or children's swing. You can also buy these bars to set up in a doorway in your home. With hands gripping the bar slightly wider than shoulder-width apart, pull yourself up toward the bar, ideally until the bar touches the top of your chest. Slowly lower and start again.

✎ Trainer's tip

The wider your grip, the more back muscle you use. Body builders often use a wide-grip chin-up to get the breadth that they need across the back.

Beginners: Ask someone to help you by holding your feet and giving you a bit of a thrust upward as you pull from the arms. As you get stronger, try coming down without their help.

Seated row

Type: Isolation exercise
Main muscles: Rhomboids

How

① Sit at a seated row machine. You may be presented with two options: either a bar requiring hands and arms to be internally rotated; or one requiring hands and arms to be externally rotated. Each will target the rhomboids in a slightly different way, so inter-change them regularly. Holding the bars, slowly pull the elbows back-wards behind the body, as far as they will go, ensuring your shoul-ders remain relaxed and depressed. Feel as though you are squeezing your shoulder blades together before releasing your arms back to their starting position again.

② **Alternative:** Tie a stretch band to a desk leg or hook it around your own feet and hold each end in your hands. Do as above with either internally or externally rotated arms.

✎ Trainer's tip

Try not to arch your lower back while doing this exercise; keep your navel pulled in towards your spine.

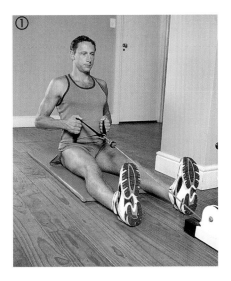

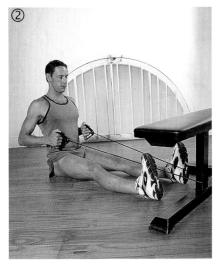

Reverse flyes

Type: Isolation exercise
Main muscles: Rhomboids

How

① Lie face down on a bench or on a corner of a bed or table. With your selected weights in each hand and keeping your hands in line with your nipples, slowly raise your hands backwards from the floor until you can feel your shoulder blades squeezing together at the top of the movement. Lower the hands back down again to the starting position.

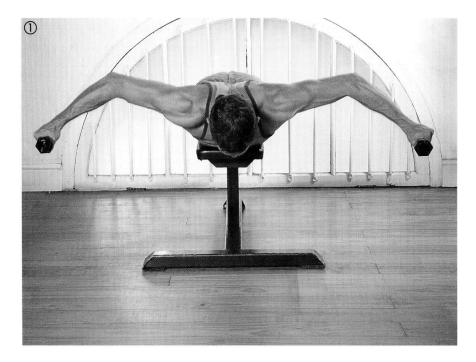

✍ Trainer's tip

Keep your shoulders depressed throughout this exercise and aim to activate the muscle highlighted in the 'hitcher' exercise (see page 62).

② **Alternative:** Hook a stretch band around the base of whatever it is you are lying on, and perform the exercise as above.

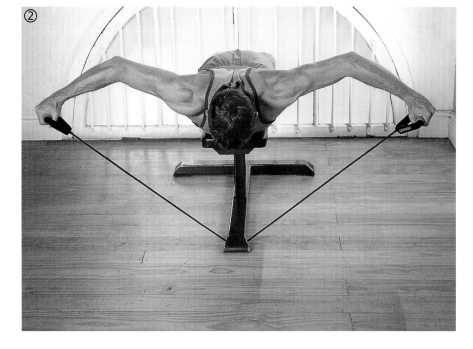

Further exercises

Suspended horizontal hyper-extension; seated back extension; chin assist

Abdominals

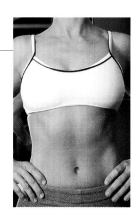

Other, more functional abdominal strengthening has already been covered in the torso stabilization section (*see* pages 60–66).

Roll-up with a twist

Type: Compound exercise
Main muscles: Rectus abdominus, internal and external obliques
Other muscles: Transversus abdominus and hip flexors, depending on your knee position

How

① Lie on your back with legs bent about 20 degrees, feet flat on the floor. With hands at your sides and just off the floor, slowly roll your body upward to about 45 degrees, twisting the torso toward the right or left at the top of the movement. Roll up one vertebra at a time – at no point should your back be flattened or arching. Refer to the 'back roll' exercise (*see* page 61) for the correct spinal position. Once you reach 45 degrees, slowly roll down again and repeat to the other side. Do this exercise very slowly to eliminate the possibility of either momentum or the hip flexors (muscles that bring the knees toward the chest) assisting your abdominals excessively.

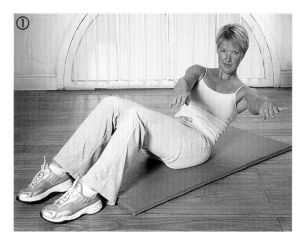

② **Beginners:** Leaving out the twisting action, start in a seated position on the floor with your legs slightly bent and arms at your sides just off the floor. Slowly lower your torso toward the floor, one vertebra at a time, until you are lying down on your back. Bend one knee into your chest and rock back up to the seated position again.

Intermediate/advanced: Fold arms across the chest (*intermediate*) or put them behind the head (*advanced*) to increase the workload on the abdominals.

🐾 Trainer's tip

The more you bend your knees, the easier this exercise becomes, as hip flexors play a bigger role when the hip joint is flexed. Avoid straightening legs to less than 20 degrees, which can be stressful on the back. Beginners can bring in some assistance by hooking a stretch band around the heels (see ③) and holding the ends in each hand while lowering to the floor.

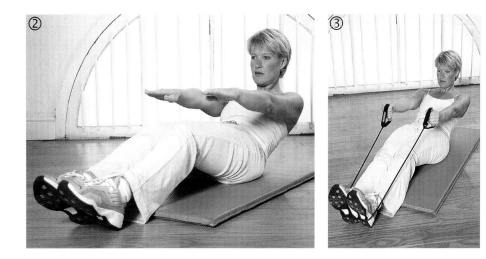

Legs and buttocks

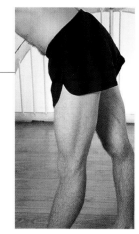

Lunges

Type: Compound exercise
Main muscles: Quadriceps (front thigh), hamstrings (back of thigh), gluteals (buttocks)

How

Stand with your feet together, hands on your hips and navel pulled to spine. Step far enough forward with one leg so that when you bend both legs you can achieve a 90-degree angle in both the front and back knees. The knee of the front foot should never fall in front of the front heel, so keep your lunge long and your weight evenly balanced between both feet. Push back to the starting point and repeat with the other leg.
Beginners: As above, but remain on one leg without stepping back in between. Bend both legs so that you achieve the same position as described above. Then straighten your working leg, repeating this several times before moving onto the other leg. This position allows you more stability, giving you the freedom to concentrate on technique instead of balance. Try holding onto something for support.
Advanced: Hold weights in your hands or place a barbell over your shoulders to increase the load on the legs.

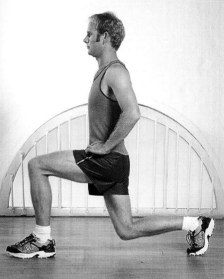

✍ Trainer's tip

Keep your chest upright and your navel pulled to your spine; avoid swinging your torso around as you step forward and back.

Side lunges

Type: Compound exercise
Main muscles: Leg adductors to pull legs toward each other into neutral position (i.e. adductor magnus, brevis and longus, gracilis muscles of inner thigh, pectineus); leg abductors to pull legs sideways away from neutral position (i.e. tensor fasciae latae, gluteus minimus)

How

Stand with legs together and hands at your sides. Keep torso upright and navel pulled toward the spine. Step out widely to one side. Keep the supporting leg straight. Bend the leg you step onto, keeping the foot facing front (parallel to the supporting foot) or slightly turned outward, if it is more comfortable. Pull the active leg back toward the start. For balance, take the arms sideways to the horizontal as you step outward.

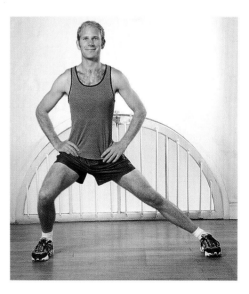

Squats

Try to perform this exercise facing forward in front of a mirror so that you can keep an eye on the position of your knees over your feet. Ideally speaking, the middle of the base of your knees should fall over the middle toe of your feet. If your knees look as though they are dropping inward (that is, falling over the big toe side of the foot), squeeze your buttocks to pull them outward. Squeeze the inner thigh if your knees are falling outward.

Type: Compound exercise

Main muscles: Quadriceps, hamstrings, gluteals

Other muscles: Erector spinae

How

① Stand with your feet slightly wider than shoulder-width apart, torso upright, navel pulled to your spine and hands at your sides. Slowly bend your knees, keeping your weight more on your heels than on your toes. Push your buttocks out to the rear as you lower yourself, while tilting your torso forward to approximately 40 degrees in order to balance your body. Raise your arms to the horizontal to help with balance.

② **Beginners:** As above, but place a chair behind you so that you can get used to lowering yourself into the correct position without the fear of unbalancing.

Advanced: As above, but work with weights in your hands, or a barbell over your shoulders.

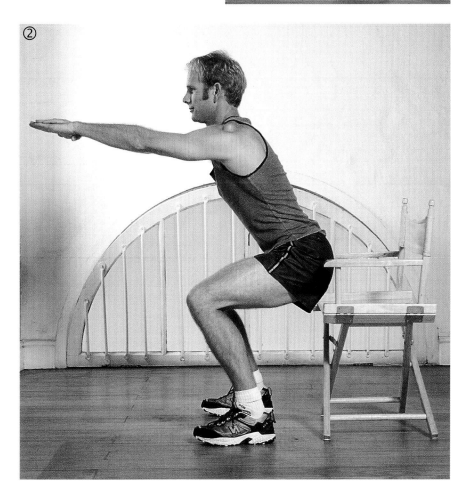

① ②

🖎 Trainer's tip

Avoid either tilting the pelvis forward or arching the lower back; and remember to keep a neutral pelvic position throughout.

Bridge

Type: Compound exercise
Main muscles: Hamstrings, gluteals, erector spinae
Other muscles: Abdominals

How

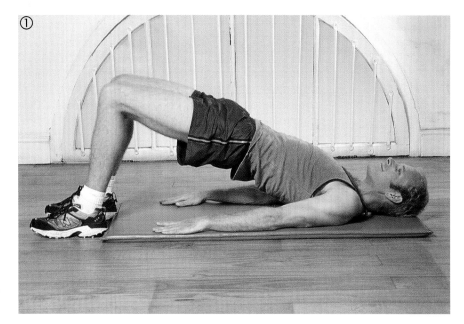

① **Beginners:** Lie on your back with feet on the floor, knees bent at a 45-degree angle and hands at your side, palms facing down. Keeping your navel pulled to your spine, slowly raise your pelvis up toward the ceiling, pushing off your feet. Aim to get your pelvis in a line with your shoulders and knees so that your body forms a diagonal line. Hold for a couple of seconds and then lower again.

② **Intermediate:** As above, but place your legs up onto a stability ball, keeping your knees bent and placed directly above your hips. Push off your calves to raise the pelvis.

③ **Advanced:** As above, but perform the exercise with one leg off the ball, held alongside the one that is on the ball.

➤ Trainer's tip

Keep your hips level, particularly if you are working on the ball with only one leg.

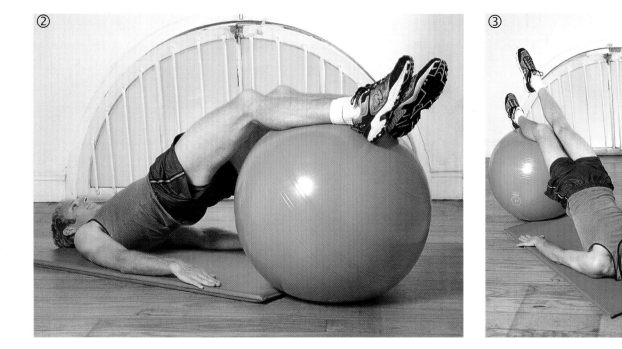

Buttock booster

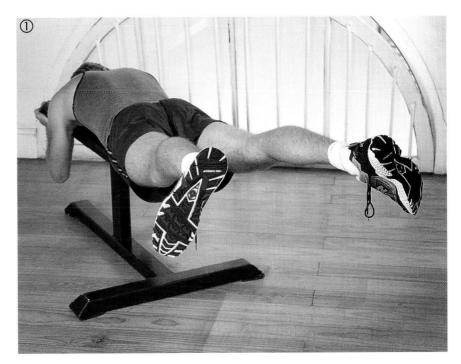

Type: Compound exercise
Main muscles: Hamstrings, gluteals, erector spinae

How

① Lie face down off the end of a narrow gym bench (or table/desk) so that your hips are only just on the bench and your feet are on the floor, if they can reach, or hanging. Hold onto the sides of the bench and slowly raise both legs, which are externally rotated, up to no more than 10 degrees above the height of your hips. Hold for a few seconds before lowering.

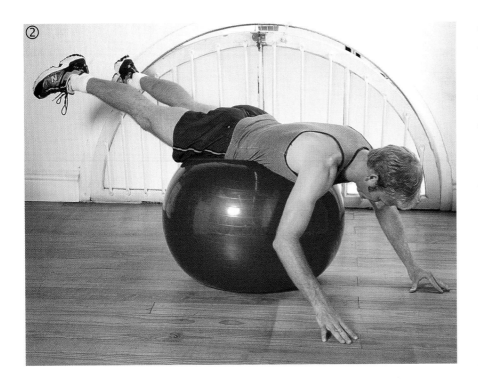

✎ Trainer's tip

While working on the ball, try to avoid shifting your body forward once you have raised the legs. This would decrease the resistance, making the exercise easier.

② **Alternative:** Do this exercise lying face down on a stability ball. Keep both hands on the floor and roll your body backwards on the ball so that it rests more on your stomach than on your thighs. Now raise the legs as above.

Further exercises

Hack squats; lying leg press; lying hamstring curl; seated leg extension; adductor machine; abductor machine

Calves

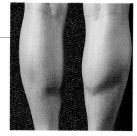

These are probably the hardest muscles to develop. If you have genetics on your side, or you have been involved in activities that use calves frequently, such as ballet, gymnastics, sprinting and synchronized swimming, you are lucky indeed. If not, these are some of the kinds of activities you could choose to become involved in to build your calf muscles.

Point and flex

Type: Compound exercise
Main muscles: Gastrocnemius, soleus, tibialis anterior
Other muscles: Quadriceps, iliopsoas

How

Either seated or standing, simply take one foot forward and point it, holding for a few seconds. Now flex the foot, again holding for a few seconds, then return to the starting position. Repeat with the other foot.

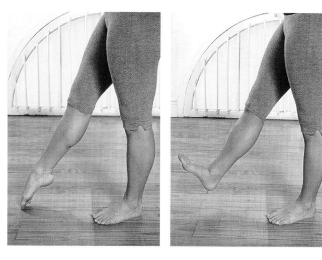

✎ Trainer's tip

Keep the knee of the working foot

straight to target both calf muscles.

Seated calf raises

Type: Isolation exercise
Main muscle: Soleus

How

Sit on a chair or in the seated calf-raise machine if you have access to one in a gym. Place your ankles directly underneath your knees. Slowly push up onto the balls of your feet to raise your knees, squeezing your calves at the top of the movement and then lowering the heels back down again. If you are using a chair, place some makeshift weights on your thighs to increase the load on the calves.

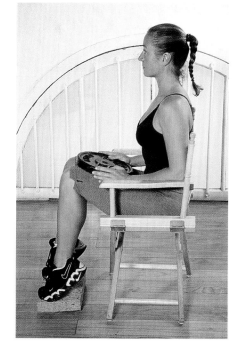

✎ Trainer's tip

If using a chair, place your feet on top of a book so there is room for the heels to hang off (if using a calf-raise machine, it will automatically allow for this heel-dropping action). Taking the calves into a stretch means that the muscle is stretched before contracting again, thus increasing the intensity of the exercise.

Standing calf raises

Type: Isolation exercise
Main muscle: Gastrocnemius

How

Use either the calf-raise machine if you have access to one in a gym or simply stand off the edge of a step and hold onto a wall for support. If standing in the machine, a load will be placed on your shoulders. Slowly rise up as high as you can onto the balls of your feet, hold for a few seconds and then lower so that your heels hang slightly off the edge of the step or foot piece, before repeating the exercise.

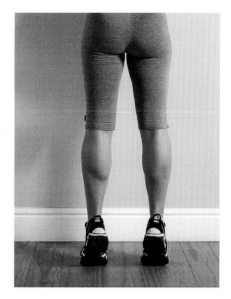

✎ *Trainer's tip*

As for seated calf raises opposite.

Flexibility training

Pectorals (chest)

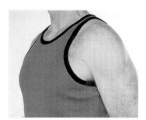

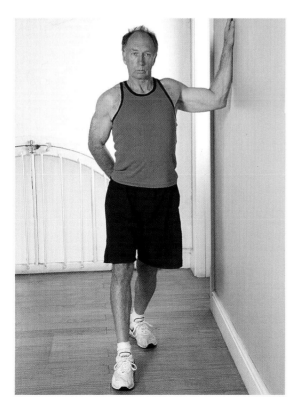

Bent-arm wall stretch

Type: Isolation stretch
Main muscle: Pectoralis major

How

Stand next to a wall with your right elbow bent at 90 degrees and your palm flat against the wall. Your elbow should be at the same height as your shoulder. Step forward onto your right foot so that your right elbow is now behind you and the stretch is felt across your chest. Ensure that your hips and shoulders remain facing the front, your navel is pulled to your spine and you maintain neutral alignment of the spine (*see* page 20). Keep shoulders down. Repeat with the left arm.

Shoulder arc

Type: Compound stretch
Main muscles: Pectoralis major and minor, deltoids

How

Seated, hold the ends of a rope or strap taut in front of you in each hand. Slowly take the arms in an arc overhead to the back of the body, keeping the elbows straight, and touching the rope or strap to the buttocks at the end of the movement. Then bring them back to the front again. Keep the stretch slow and controlled, as you are potentially putting the shoulder into a vulnerable position in the third quarter of this arc. Do not allow your ribs to stick out or your back to arch.

Alternative: Stand with your arms behind your chest, your hands clasped, ensuring that your shoulders do not roll forward.

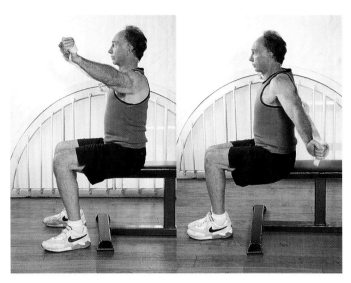

✍ Trainer's tip

At first, if your shoulders are very tight, you will probably need to hold the rope with your hands fairly far apart in order to be able to take the arms behind you. As you become looser, try to move your hands closer toward one another.

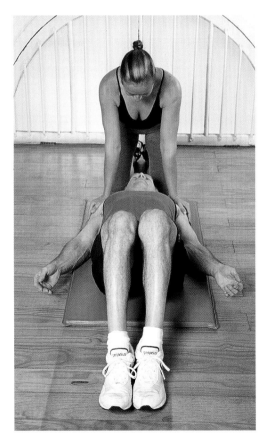

Open chest press

You will need a partner for this one.
Type: Isolation stretch
Main muscle: Pectoralis minor

How

Lie down on your back on the floor, with your arms at your sides and your palms facing upward. Ask someone to kneel at your head and cup the front of your shoulders with their hands, so that they are pushing down on your shoulders from above. You should feel a good stretch across the front of your shoulders as well as into your chest.

Alternative: Lie on a towel rolled up and placed along the length of the spine, as this will serve to open up the chest further. You can do this without a partner, or with a partner as in the exercise above if you want increase the stretch.

Deltoids (shoulder muscles)

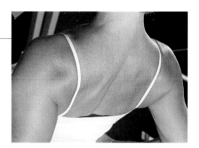

Elbow up, elbow down

Type: Compound stretch
Main muscles: Tricep of the top arm, anterior deltoid of lower arm

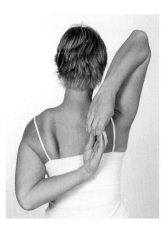

How

Sit or stand with the spine in neutral alignment. Take your right arm behind your back with the palm facing away from your back and bend the elbow so that your fingers point up your spine. Stretch your left arm up to the ceiling, bend the elbow and bring the hand down with the palm facing your back to clasp the right hand. Keep your ribs tucked in and open up your chest; do not allow the shoulder of the lower arm to roll forward. Try to flatten the armpit of your raised arm and keep your elbow close to your ear, pointing up toward the ceiling. Your lower arm should be as close to the body as possible. Avoid allowing a space between your waist and elbow. Repeat on the other side.

Strap stretch

Type: Compound exercise
Main muscles: Triceps, posterior deltoid

How

Measure a rope or strap so that a loop in it is equivalent to your shoulder width. Place the loop around your elbows and then kneel in front of a bench or bed so that your knees are directly underneath your hips and your elbows are resting on the edge of the bench or bed.
① **Beginners:** Clasp your hands together, keeping them directly above your elbows. Slowly try to get your head and neck into line with your spine, which should be in neutral alignment.
② **Intermediate/advanced:** As above, but place a book or ball between your wrists, not your hands, and keep your hands directly above the elbows (see below left). The book or ball should keep your hands sufficiently open, but not wider than your elbows.

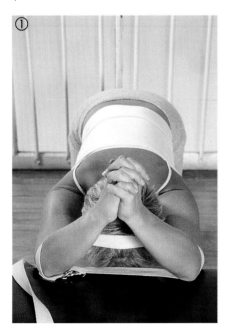

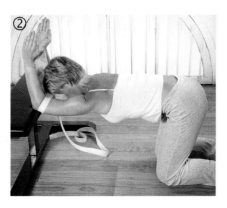

✎ Trainer's tip

If your shoulders are very tight, strap your elbows further apart rather than close together.

Arms

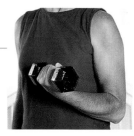

Straight-arm wall stretch

Type: Compound stretch
Main muscles: Biceps, pectorals

How

Stand next to a wall with your left arm extended backwards as near to shoulder height as you can, and the back of your hand against the wall so your arm is internally rotated. Step forward onto your right foot until the stretch is felt in the bicep. If you are particularly tight in the front body, you may also feel it across your chest. Ensure that your hips and shoulders remain facing the front. Repeat on the other side.

✍ Trainer's tip

Try as far as possible to keep your shoulders down.

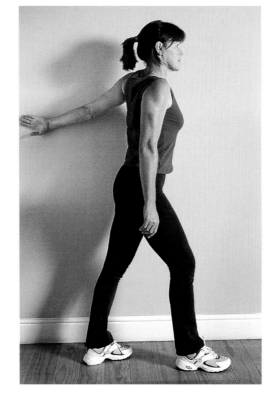

Elbow up

Type: Isolation stretch
Main muscle: Triceps

How

Either sit or stand with your spine in neutral alignment. Stretch your left arm up to the ceiling, then bend your elbow and bring your hand down, with the palm facing your back. Try to flatten your armpit and keep your elbow close to your ear, pointing up toward the ceiling. Hold the elbow with your right hand and pull it gently toward your left ear. Repeat the exercise on the other side.

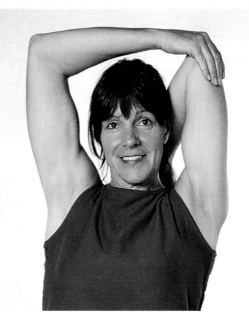

Back

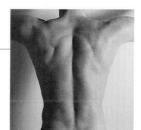

Forward curl

Type: Isolation stretch
Main muscle: Erector spinae

How

How: Sit back on your heels with your feet on the floor, so that your feet are together and your knees apart. Keep your hands at your sides and drop your head down to rest on the floor in front of your knees, resting on your forehead.

Alternative: The same stretch can be done lying on your back. Simply hug your bent knees in toward your chest.

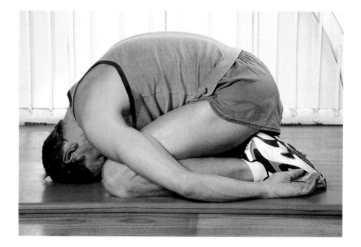

Straight-arm forward curl

Type: Compound stretch
Main muscles: Latissimus dorsi, teres major, rhomboids, mid-trapezius, posterior deltoid

How

As with the 'forward curl' stretch above, but this time extend your arms so that they are straight and above your head, with palms flat on the floor. Try to push your chest toward the floor.

Alternative: Stand in front of a desk or any piece of equipment you can use to hold onto so that you are leaning forward, with your back at 90 degrees to your legs. Push your chest gently downward toward the floor, bending your knees slightly. Keep your head in line with your spine.

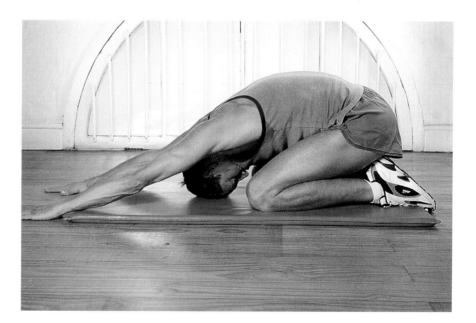

Hand over knee

Type: Compound stretch
Main muscles: Rhomboids, middle trapezius

How

Sit on a bench or bed with your knees bent and legs apart. Place each hand around the outside of the opposite knee (right hand around left knee and vice versa). Drop your head down and bend the top of your torso forward as you pull your knees apart. You should feel this stretch across your middle back.

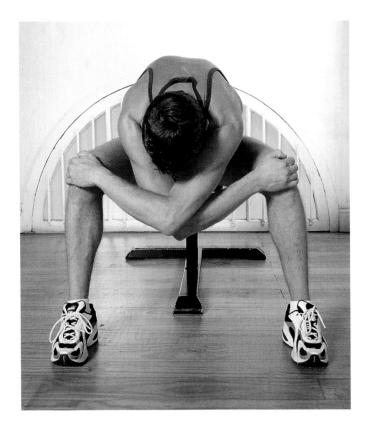

Thoracic release

Type: Isolation stretch
Main muscles: Erectus spinae
This is a good release for people who have tight upper backs (hunched or stooped). It also opens up the chest at the same time.

How

Lie on your back and place a short, tightly rolled towel, folded double, between your shoulder blades so that your head and shoulders rest on the floor but your chest is raised off it. Keep legs straight, with knees together and hands on the floor at your sides.

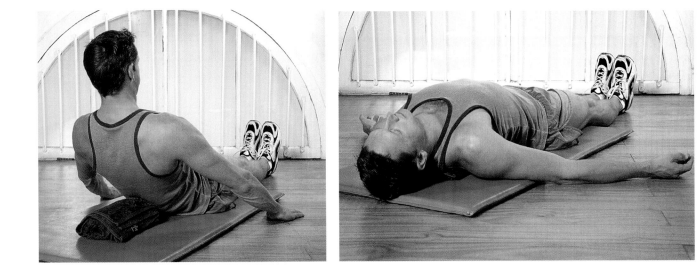

Abdominals

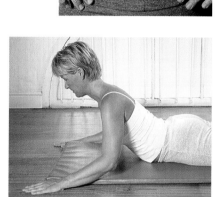

Cobra

Type: Isolation stretch
Main muscle: Rectus abdominus

How

Lie on your stomach on the floor with your hands in front of your shoulders, elbows bent and palms facing down. Slowly lift your torso off the ground up to approximately 45 degrees. Once you are at the top of this movement, breathe in and try to push your stomach out so that you feel a stretch across it. Breathe out as you lower again.

Elevated back bend

Type: Compound stretch
Main muscles: Abdominals, iliopsoas

How

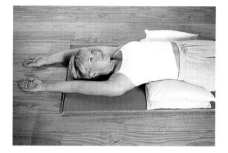

Lie on your back and place two pillows or cushions under your sacrum (the area below your lumbar spine and above your coccyx). This should raise your pelvis enough for you to feel a mild stretch into your abdominal area. Keep your legs straight and together. To increase the stretch, take your arms overhead. Should you experience lower-back pain when doing this, however, keep your hands at your sides.

Standing side stretch

Type: Compound
Main muscles: Obliques, quadratus lumborum (lower back), latissimus dorsi (mid back), teres major (mid/upper back), triceps

How

Stand squarely and clasp your hands above your head, with your elbows straight and your palms facing each other. Keeping your navel pulled toward your spine to support the lower back, slowly lean over to the right, as far as you can go, stretching your hands towards the right. Repeat the exercise on the other side.

✎ Trainer's tip

Aim to lengthen your spine while performing this stretch. Also ensure that your chest and shoulders face directly forward, with the top arm directly over your top ear rather than in front of it.

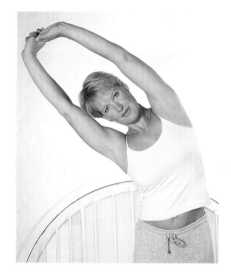

Legs and buttocks

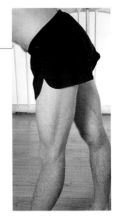

Seated hamstring

If your hamstrings are very tight, you may find this exercise uncomfortable. Do the 'lying hamstring' stretch below instead.
Type: Compound stretch
Main muscles: Hamstrings, gastrocnemius

How

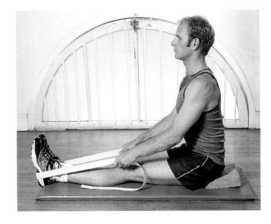

Sit on a firm cushion on the floor with your legs extended in front of your body. Pull the flesh of your buttocks backwards out from under your 'sitting' bones so that your pelvis is in a neutral position – that is, your lower back has a slight arch (not shown here). Hook a strap around your heels, hold on to the ends with both hands and, keeping the neutral position, slowly take the front of your chest towards your feet. Keep your feet flexed, your thigh muscles pulled up and your knees straight and facing the ceiling.

✑ Trainer's tip

If you want to increase the calf stretch in both of the exercises on this page, place the strap around the balls of your feet instead of around your heels. The more you bring your toes back toward your chest, the more you will increase the stretch in the calves.

Lying hamstring

Type: Compound stretch
Main muscles: Hamstrings, gastrocnemius

How

Lie on your back on the floor with both legs extended. Bend one leg and place a strap around the heel of that leg. Holding both ends in your hands, slowly raise your heel up to the ceiling, straightening the knee of your raised leg. You are aiming eventually for a 90-degree angle between this leg and the floor. The knee of the leg on the floor should also remain straight and should be facing the ceiling with the thigh contracted. This leg anchors the body and will ensure that the pelvis remains in neutral alignment instead of rolling into a posterior tilt (*see* page 20), as it is inclined to do in this position. Repeat with the other leg.

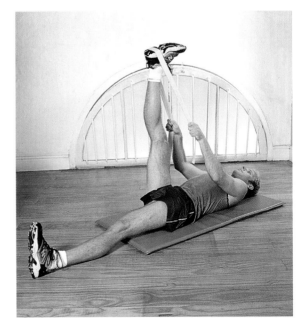

Standing thigh stretch

Type: Compound stretch
Main muscles: Quadriceps, iliopsoas

How

Stand and hold your left foot behind you and against your left buttock with your left hand. Keep your right leg straight and support yourself with your right hand against a wall or chair. Pull your navel toward your spine and ensure that your knees are joined (side by side) as you gently push your pubic bone forward and lengthen your spine. Repeat on the other side.

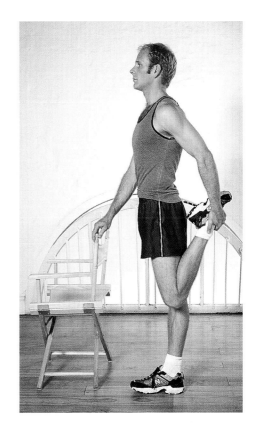

Foot over knee

Type: Compound stretch
Main muscles: The muscles that outwardly rotate the hip (i.e. the piriformis, gemellus superior and inferior, obturator externus and internus, quadratus femoris, gluteus maximus – all in the buttocks)

How

Lie on your back with your left leg bent, foot flat on the floor. Place your right foot onto your left knee with the foot flexed. Take your right arm between your legs, your left arm around the outside of your left leg and clasp both over the left knee, pulling it upward toward your chest. If you find it difficult to keep your head down on the floor, put a pillow underneath it. Try to relax the upper body and breathe through the stretch. Avoid leaning your raised knee and body toward the right, as this reduces the stretch; rather try to keep your body as straight as possible while pulling your left knee in as close to the chest as possible. Repeat on the other side.

Alternative: This stretch can be done with the left foot resting on a wall and knee bent at 90 degrees. Place your right knee as above and gently press downwards on it with your right hand to intensify the stretch.

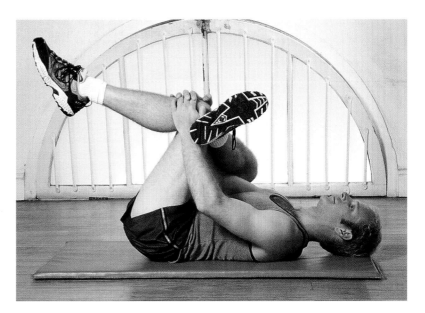

Butterfly

Type: Compound stretch
Main muscles: Muscles around the pelvis (gracilis, pectineus, tensor fascia latae, gluteus medius and minimus) that internally rotate the thighs, as well as those that pull the legs together (adductors)

How

Sit on the floor on a firm cushion or folded towel with the bottom of your feet touching one another and your knees bent and dropped outward to the sides. Pull the flesh of your buttocks backwards out from under your 'sitting' bones so that your pelvis is in a neutral position. Hold your ankles with your hands and lean your elbows onto your knees, pushing them down gently.

Alternative: This exercise can be done lying on your back to increase the stretch across the pelvis. Be careful, however, not to arch the lower back excessively.

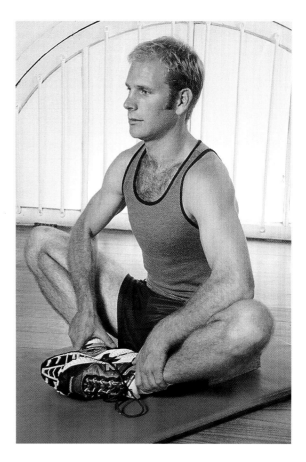

Stride

Type: Compound stretch
Main muscles: Leg adductors that pull the legs together (i.e. adductor magnus, brevis and longus of the inner thigh, as well as the pectineus, which lies in front of the pubis)

How

Sit on the floor on a firm cushion or folded towel, with your legs straight and opened to the sides. Pull the flesh of your buttocks backwards out from under your 'sitting' bones so that your pelvis is in a neutral position. Holding your calves with your hands, gently move your chest toward the floor between your feet, keeping your spine elongated. Ensure that your feet point upward to the ceiling at all times.

✍ Trainer's tip

If you experience pain on the inside of your knee during this exercise, your legs may be too wide apart.

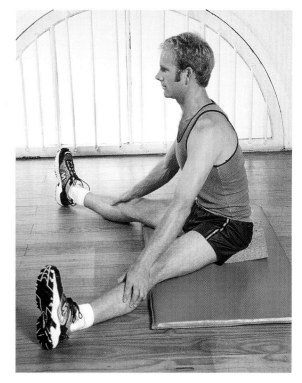

Calves

Heel dip

Type: Isolation stretch
Main muscle: Gastrocnemius

How

Stand with the right foot on a raised object or step, and the heel of the left foot hanging off the edge of the same object or step, both feet parallel to one another. Support yourself with a hand on the wall. Slightly bend the right knee and slowly lower the left heel until you feel a stretch in your calf. Repeat on the other side.

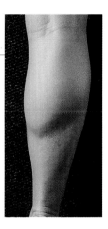

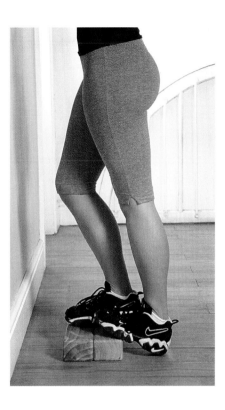

✎ Trainer's tip

Keep both your shoulders slightly forward of your hips and your abdominals activated, as this will ensure that you do not arch your lower back.

Bent-knee calf stretch

Type: Isolation stretch
Main muscle: Soleus

How

Stand on both feet, one placed about a foot behind the other. Keeping your weight on your back foot and feet parallel to one another, bend both knees until you feel a stretch in the calf of your back leg. Repeat on the other side.

✎ Trainer's tip

Keep shoulders slightly forward of your hips and ensure that your feet are not placed too far away from each other. Keeping them close together ensures that the weight of your body offers a deep stretch.

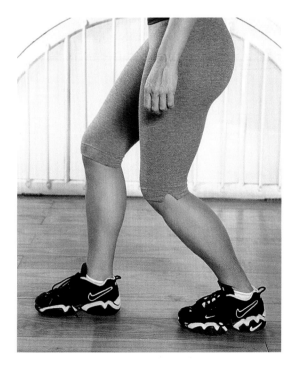

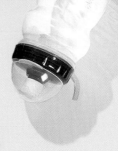

Good things to Know

In the first two chapters, you learned how to decide on your personal health and fitness goals, and how to assess your fitness level and motivation. In the next two, we looked at the general principles of effective exercise before moving onto the main menu – that is, to the exercises themselves. To conclude, let us look briefly at some related issues.

The right gear

Shoes are arguably the most important aspect of workout gear, and it is vital that you wear the right ones for your chosen activity. Most sports shops that sell a wide range of training shoes should have knowledgeable sales staff to give you sound advice. Since trainers are with you for a long time and can be expensive, always visit a couple of stores to get a second opinion before you make your purchase.

It is advisable to have your foot and your walking or running style evaluated. Contact a chiropodist or podiatrist for advice on who to go

to; the best would be a specialist who deals specifically with physical activity or sport-related stances, as opposed to general posture.

Shoes are specifically designed for different activities.
Running shoes have lots of cushioning in the heel, as this is the first part of your foot to strike the ground, although many off-road running shoes have all-over cushioning.
Aerobics shoes have more toe cushioning, as you work through from the balls of your feet first in this type of activity. They also offer underfoot traction for additional grip on studio floors.
Hiking shoes have more ankle stability to protect you when walking on uneven terrain, while *walking shoes* should offer general stability and comfort.
Cross trainers have all-over cushioning for people engaging in a number of different activities.

Ensure that the shoes you settle on are both comfortable and appropriate for your activity.

When choosing **socks**, make comfort your priority. Those made

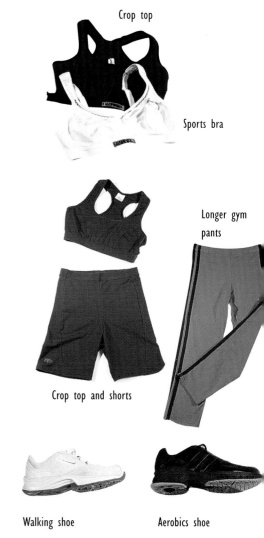

Crop top

Sports bra

Longer gym pants

Crop top and shorts

Walking shoe

Aerobics shoe

from natural fabrics, such as cotton, or moisture-management fabrics are best, since they help to absorb sweat. Note, though, that cotton also tends to hold sweat, whereas treated fabrics carry it to the surface to allow for increased evaporation. Seamless socks with added toe cushioning are excellent for minimizing your exposure to blisters. Some socks offer arch support to keep the foot secure during vigorous activity, such as aerobics.

Clothing is often selected on personal taste, although some environmental issues need to be considered. It may seem fairly obvious, but if you are working out on a really hot day, try to wear clothes that are loose-fitting and light, and preferably short in the sleeves and legs. If training outdoors in sunny weather, wear a peak cap and sun protection. The use of caps is to be discouraged indoors, even if it is trendy, since you lose a lot of heat from your head and wearing a cap slows down the cooling process.

In very cold weather, warmer fabrics with longer sleeves and legs are good. A cap would also work well to hold some of your heat while you warm up.

In terms of fabric types, it is a good idea to wear stretch fabrics for any physical activity that requires you to bend joints frequently. Picture yourself at a kick boxing class in a pair of jeans and you will see the logic of this. Alternatively, if you prefer non-stretch fabrics, keep your workout gear to shorts of knee or mid-thigh length.

While cotton is a comfortable natural fibre that absorbs sweat well, it also holds it well, which means that you may stay wet while exercising. Unless you perspire heavily, this should not be too much of a problem; if you do, you may want to consider synthetic nylon/spandex fabric that dries quickly so is useful for longer workouts. It is used by many

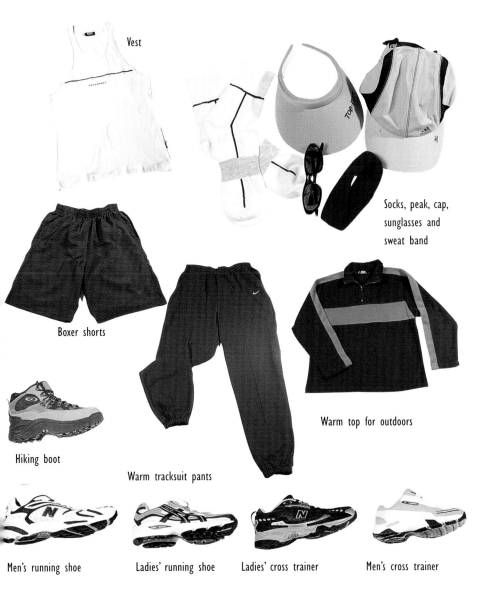

Vest

Socks, peak, cap, sunglasses and sweat band

Boxer shorts

Warm top for outdoors

Hiking boot

Warm tracksuit pants

Men's running shoe

Ladies' running shoe

Ladies' cross trainer

Men's cross trainer

Left: Being comfortable in your training gear can make a big difference to how you experience your workout.

serious athletes and recreational sportspeople – for example, you may have noticed cycling shorts made from this shiny fabric.

Some moisture-management fabrics have been treated with a finish that mimics natural fabric in terms of sweat absorption but it dries really quickly too. It does this by drawing perspiration to the surface of the fabric where it can evaporate effectively. Apart from these treated fabrics, other specially constructed fabrics exist that provide the same effect.

Relatively new are anti-bacterial fabrics, which can be useful when you are unable to shower immediately after your workout and need to spend a few hours in sweaty gear. If you have ever been in this situation, you may have experienced the itchiness or discomfort that comes with fungal infections.

All of the fabrics already mentioned are available in stretch and non-stretch versions, so it is best to make your decision according to your chosen activity.

In addition, new-generation synthetics called Microfibres, also in combination with spandex, are coming onto the market. Apart from feeling more luxurious against the skin, they have enhanced moisture-management properties.

For those people exercising outdoors, particularly in cool weather, a rip-stop fabric like that used for making parachutes can be used for its warmth and light weight. Although it is tightly woven to prevent too much air passing through, it is permeable – and is therefore breathable.

In general, use the rule of comfort to guide your decisions here – if your clothing is restrictive in any way, you are unlikely to achieve an optimal workout.

Another item of clothing some women may want to consider is a sports bra. Here are some things to look out for when making your selection.

- Comfort is paramount.
- For full support, choose a bra with a broad band across the back and wide shoulder straps.
- Avoid bras with too many clips or hooks, which can chafe.
- Choose a cotton bra, or one with a high percentage of cotton, which is comfortable on the skin and allows it to breathe.

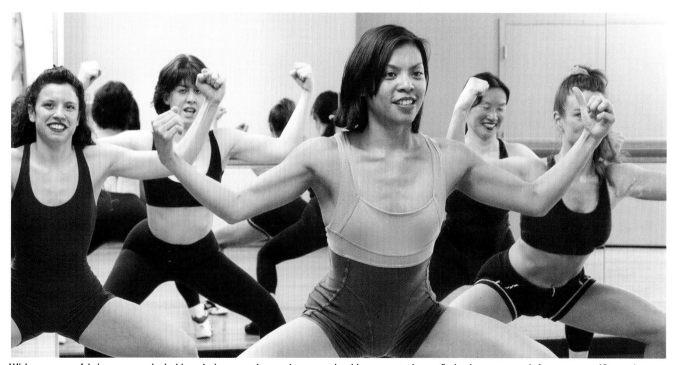

With so many fabric types and clothing designs on the market, you should not struggle to find what you need for your specific workout.

Hydration

Drinking water at regular intervals throughout your workout makes a water bottle an essential access-ory. Do not rely on thirst as an indicator because you are often already dehydrated by the time you feel thirsty. A good indica-tor of a hydrated body is pale yellow or clear urine; dark yellow urine shows dehyd-ration. Bear in mind that coffee, tea and alcohol are all diuretics that dehydrate the body, even though your urine may appear to be clear.

The American College of Sports Medicine (ACSM) recommends a fluid intake of 230–340ml (8–12 fl oz) 15 minutes before your exer-cise session; 85–115ml (3–4 fl oz) every 10 to 15 minutes during your session; 450ml (16 fl oz) for every 5kg (11lb) of weight lost during the session. This means that you should weigh yourself before and after your workout to determine general fluid loss. Do this a couple of times to get an idea of an average figure.

The ACSM also recommends that for any physical activity session of less than 60 minutes, water is an adequate and, in fact, desirable fluid replacement. For a workout longer than 60 minutes, sports drinks may be beneficial, since they supply energy and electrolytes, and encourage further fluid intake. If you are dehydrated, you will find that you fatigue more quickly and may lose co-ordination too. When choosing your sports drink, here are some things you may want to consider.

- Do not exceed a 10 per cent carbohydrate solution; most sports drinks offer about a 6–8 per cent solution.
  - Make sure the tempera-ture of the drink is to your liking. If you prefer it cold, make a plan to keep it that way until you start your workout.
  - Choose a drink that offers electrolytes, but not in vast quantities, as these will make the drink salty and therefore unpalatable.
  - Avoid drinks that are too sweet as these are unlikely to quench your thirst.
- Taste is important; the fact is that if you do not enjoy it, it is unlikely you will drink it.
- If you prefer a taste-free drink, use a glucose polymer solution.

Measuring heart rate

It is important and useful to know your *resting heart rate (pulse)*, as this will tell you how efficiently your heart pumps blood around your body when at rest. Generally speaking, the lower this figure is the fitter your heart is. An average range is between 70 and 90 beats per minute. If your resting pulse happens to be lower than the average but you do not actually do any exercise, give this book to someone who really needs it! Seriously, this means your heart is naturally quite efficient at pumping your blood around your body: for the same amount of blood needed by your body, your heart beats fewer times, thus reducing its workload, since each beat is powerful enough to deliver a greater volume of blood.

To take your resting pulse, place the first two fingers of your right hand on your wrist just below the base of your left thumb. You will see a slight hollow over which you can

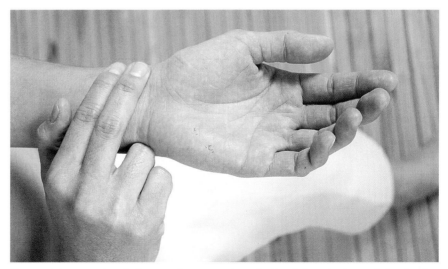

Measure heart rate by placing two fingers on the wrist just below the base of the thumb.

place your fingers. Count the beats for a full minute. Do this first thing in the morning before you get out of bed, preferably for three days consecutively for an average reading.

As you get fitter, your resting pulse starts to drop – an indication that your heart is becoming stronger and more efficient.

It is equally useful to measure your pulse during your exercise session. This measurement tells you how well, or not, your heart is coping, giving you the opportunity either to increase your workout intensity if your heart rate is too low, or to decrease it if your heart rate is too high. There are three ways to measure exercise intensity: by taking your pulse manually, by means of a heart rate monitor, and by a perceived scale of exertion.

Taking your pulse *manually* while working out requires you to stop your activity in order to be able to feel your heart beat. Try to find your pulse within five seconds of stopping. Instead of counting for a full minute, you could take it for 15 seconds and multiply by four to give you a figure over a minute. For example, if your 15-second reading gives you a figure of 26, multiply it by four. Your pulse is therefore 104 beats per minute.

Using a *heart rate monitor* is an easy way to see how your heart is coping without having to fumble around for a pulse. Most monitors require you to place a transmitter band around your chest, just below your nipple line. The belt reads your pulse and transmits it as a per-minute figure to a receiver

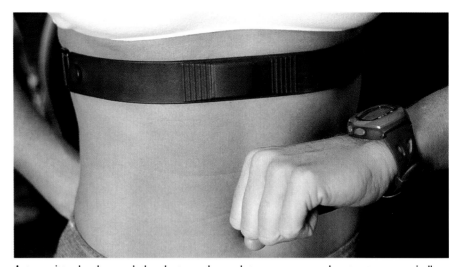

A transmitter band around the chest can be used to measure your heart rate automatically.

worn as a watch around your wrist. Base decisions to increase, maintain or decrease your intensity on the figure displayed on the watch.

Using a *perceived scale of exertion* helps you connect more with what you are feeling than what your pulse is reading. Use the table on the right for an effective means of gauging intensity. Although it may seem a little abstract at first, the more you work with it, the more accurate you will become. It is a useful tool if you struggle to find your pulse in a hurry, or do not want to buy a heart rate monitor, which can be quite expensive.

To know whether or not you are working at the right intensity, you need to predetermine what your goals are, and thus how hard you need to work. Once you have taken your resting heart rate, apply the following formula to determine what your maximum heart rate is – in other words, the hardest your heart can work:

Males: 220 – age (in years) = maximum heart rate
Females: 226 – age (in years) = maximum heart rate

CATEGORY-RATIO SCALE OF PERCEIVED EXERTION

0	Nothing at all	No intensity
0.3		
0.5	Extremely weak	Just noticeable
0.7		
1	Very weak	Light
1.5		
2	Weak	Light
2.5		
3	Moderate	
4		
5	Strong	Heavy
6		
7	Very strong	
8		
9		
10	Extremely strong	Strongest intensity
11		
*	Absolute maximum	Highest possible

Source: ACSM

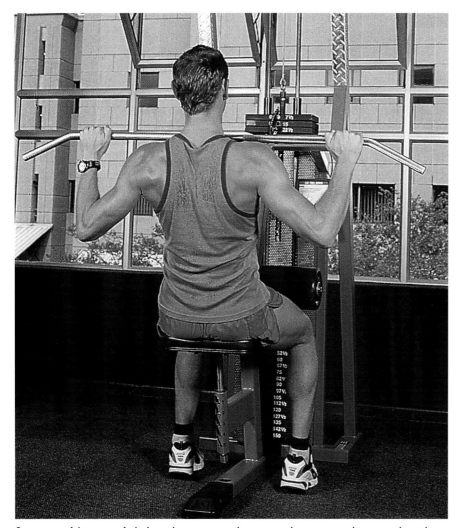

Be aware of how you feel throughout an exercise so you learn to monitor your intensity.

Once you are comfortable at a moderate intensity, start to include some *high-intensity* activity (between 85 and 95 per cent).

Using the maximum figure you worked out from the formula, multiply it by your chosen intensity percentage to work out your actual figure, expressed in beats per minute (bpm). Here is an example:

As a woman, aged 26, your maximum heart rate is (226–26) x 200bpm. You are a beginner to exercise so you choose to work at between 60 and 75 per cent of your maximum heart rate. Thus, 200 x 60 per cent = 120bpm and 200 x 75 per cent = 150bpm. Therefore, the range of heart rates within which you should be working is 120 to 150bpm. If your pulse is higher than that during your workout – or, if you are using perceived exertion, should you feel that you are working harder than the top of this range – adjust your effort accordingly. Apply the reverse if your pulse is dropping below the bottom of the range.

As you become more used to equating heart rate with how you feel during a workout, it becomes easier to make the necessary adjustments in intensity without having to measure the heart rate.

Bear in mind that this formula is a generalized one, so you may be able to work above your so-called maximum, or you may be unable to reach this figure. To be on the safe side, use this formula as your guide.

In order for cardiovascular fitness to improve, you should try to train somewhere between 60 and 90 per cent of your maximum heart rate. It is recommended that you start at a *low intensity* of between 55 and 70 per cent of your maximum heart rate, then gradually build up to a *moderate intensity* of between 70 and 85 per cent over a period of six to 14 weeks, assuming regular physical activity is taking place.

	INTENSITY OF ACTIVITY		
	LOW	**MODERATE**	**HIGH**
Maximum heart rate	**55%–70%**	**70%–85%**	**85%–95%**

Demystifying the gym

There seem to be two types of people in this world – those who go to gym, and those who do not! This is not to say that if you do not belong to a gym you are not active; in fact, many people would far rather exercise outdoors – in the mountains or on the beach, for instance – than in a stuffy, crowded and unnatural environment. Nonetheless, there are many people who enjoy the energy in a gym, the social aspect, as well as the opportunity to do everything within one environment. It does not follow, though, that those who go to gym are necessarily particularly active. Plenty of gym members walk in, mess around half-heartedly with some form of exercise and then sit in the sauna or juice bar for the greater part of their time there.

If you already go to the gym regularly, skip the next section, which is specifically for those who want to join a gym, but are unsure about what to do and how to do it.

Gym etiquette

Believe it or not, there is such a thing as gym etiquette. Most gyms have a set of rules and regulations to which you are asked to adhere. Together with the most common of these, here are some of the unspoken rules:

• **Do** wear trainers while working out – you do not want to lose a big toe in the pit (which is gym lingo for weights area).

• **Do** use a towel at all times – no one else wants to work in your sweat, nor do you want to work directly on a piece of equipment that has been used by 30,000 other sweaty people before you.

• **Do** respect designated areas in the gym – keep weights in the pit; perform cardiovascular activities in the appropriate area; stretch in the mat area (gyms usually offer a fair amount of space for toning and stretching activities); and swim in the pool, etc.

• **Do** pack your weights away when you have finished – you will find racks for sets of barbells and dumbbells in the pit, so make sure you put them back in the right spot.

• **Do** wait in the queue for cardio equipment – most gyms will allow you a set amount of time on each machine during peak hours. You are likely to find out just how big and strong muscles can get if you try to jump this queue or stay too long on one piece of equipment!

• **Do** feel free to complain about any dissatisfaction you may have with the gym's environment or service – suggestion cards are often at the front desk. Things that may irritate you include music level and type, unfriendly staff, equipment in disrepair, and inattentive instructors.

• **Do not** swear or use sexist, racist or abusive language – even if your foot is under a 200kg dumbbell.

• **Do not** fill your water bottle at the drinking fountain while there is a queue behind you – wait till it is quiet, or walk to the nearest bathroom for a top-up.

• **Do not** laugh at anyone else while they are exercising – they may have a good reason to be seated backwards on the rowing machine. You never know.

• **Do not** try to 'hit on' anyone while they are training. You are all there to work out. (Well, that is what fitness practitioners like to believe anyway.)

Gym lingo

To help you understand what the Neanderthal next to you is saying when he grunts, 'Uh – come over here and spot my last rep of hammy curls,' and make you appear more knowledgeable when speaking 'gym talk', some words you need to know are listed in the table below:

GYM TALK

Spot – *assist*

Pecs – *pectoral muscles*

Abs – *abdominal muscles*

Delts – *deltoid muscles*

Tris (pronounced 'trize') – *triceps*

Bis (pronounced 'bize') – *biceps*

Quads – *quadriceps*

Hams/hammys – *hamstrings*

Glutes – *gluteal muscles*

Lats – *latissimus dorsi muscles*

Traps – *trapezius muscles*

Reps – *repetitions*

Sets – *groups of repetitions*

What can I expect from fitness staff?

Almost all gyms will employ the services of a gym or floor instructor. They are often referred to as the 'packers and stackers', since they are required to keep the gym free of clutter – that is, weights and other accessories that people have left lying all over the floor. They are also there to assist members, and although their qualifications do not necessarily allow them to develop individual programmes, they should be able to provide you with some sound training advice. They should definitely know enough to come over and tell you when you are facing the wrong way on a machine.

A gym may also offer the services of a personal trainer. Whether or not you are required to pay extra for such a service depends on gym policy. Personal trainers can be great motivators for newcomers, since they require you to book sessions with them ahead of time, thus ensuring that your workout time is scheduled in your diary. They also have skills and knowledge that enable them to develop a personalized and therefore effective programme for a client. Since they will screen and assess you before starting a working relationship, they will have insight into your history and current exercise and health status, as well as your unique goals and objectives. They can assist you in developing an action plan, which will help you remain focused and motivated. Before taking on a trainer, however, be sure to ask a couple of key questions.

1. *Are you qualified?*
   Find out when the personal trainer qualified; if it was 30 years ago, and he or she has not done any courses since then, you may want to reconsider.
2. *Are you licensed to practise?*
   Some countries require fitness practitioners to be licensed with a council. This way, a nationally acceptable standard is applied. If they are not required to do so, find out if your prospective trainer is a member of a fitness registration body.

3. *Have you completed any further education since qualifying?*
   Since the fitness industry offers new insights into training on a regular basis, it makes sense that those with integrity remain as up to date as possible on these findings. Ideally, they should have completed at least one seminar, workshop or course every year since qualifying.

Below: Get assistance if you think you may struggle with technique or weight.

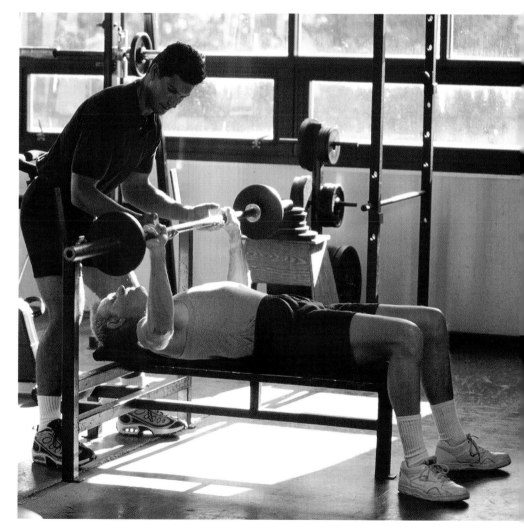

Gym Machines

Gym equipment

Gym equipment can be fairly daunting, even to those who have trained in the fitness environment for years. To help you understand how such equipment should be used, some of the most commonly found machines are illustrated on the following pages, together with an explanation of which parts of the body they are intended to train.

Bear in mind that different pieces of equipment or gym systems are used by different gyms, so sometimes a piece of equipment for the same body part can be presented in a different way. For example, the bench press exercise can be done either seated or lying down. Generally, though, the information given in the following pages should give you a pretty good idea of what is expected of you when using the equipment.

Pectorals (chest)

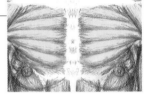

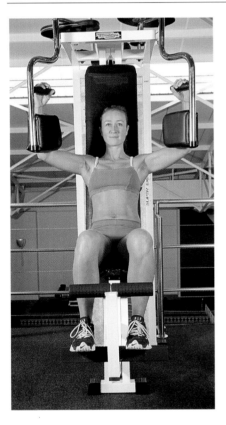

↶ PEC DECK

Sit facing outward, and place your forearms onto the pads so that your elbows are at shoulder height, hands directly above them. Place your feet on the footrest and lean your back against the backrest. Now squeeze your elbows as close together as possible before releasing back to the starting position, ensuring that your elbows stay in line with or slightly in front of your chest. If you find this too difficult, even on the lightest weight plate, drop your elbows so that you are holding the pads with your hands instead of your forearms.

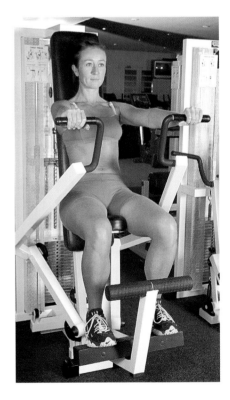

SEATED BENCH PRESS ↷

Sit facing away from the machine with your back leaning against the backrest. Place your feet up onto the footrest and take hold of the grips with your hands, slowly pushing them forward until your arms straighten before releasing them back down to your starting position. You may find that you need to push down onto the additional footplate in order to move the hand grips a little away from the body before you start this exercise.

Shoulders

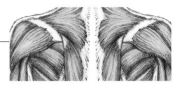

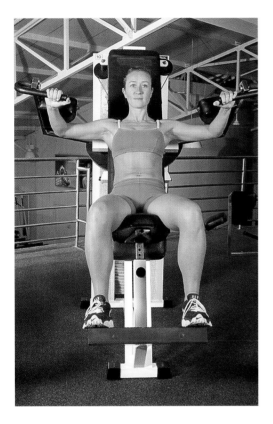

⟲ SIDE RAISE

Sit facing away from the machine with your feet on the footplate. The seat height can usually be adjusted to suit your body. With bent arms, take hold of the grips with your hands and lean your elbows against the padded arm. Slowly raise your arms out to your sides and then back down to the starting point again. Be sure to keep your shoulders depressed throughout this exercise. Sometimes these machines have an additional footplate that gives you the opportunity to manoeuvre the handgrips into a more comfortable starting position.

SHOULDER PRESS ⟱

Sit facing away from the machine with your back leaning against the backrest. The seat is usually adjustable to suit your height. Place your feet on the footplate and hold the grips with your hands. Slowly raise your arms until they straighten, then return to the starting position. Sometimes this machine will offer you either a narrow or wide grip: the narrower it is, the more front deltoid muscle you use; the wider, the more side deltoid. As with the side-raise machine, the shoulder press may provide you with an additional footplate that gives you the opportunity to manoeuvre the hand grips into a more comfortable starting position.

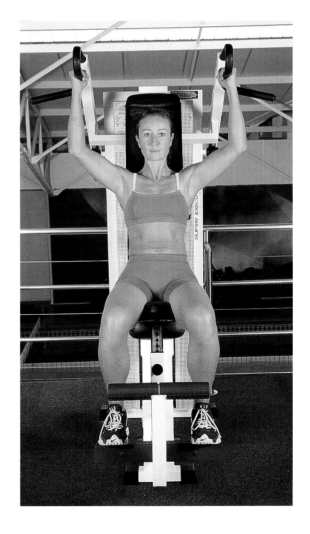

Arms

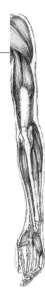

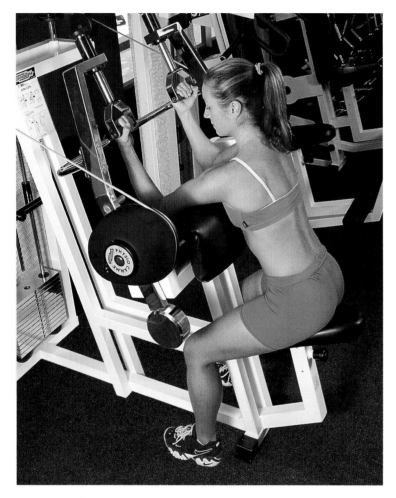

BICEP CURL

Sit facing the machine with your feet squarely on the floor and your elbows resting on the arm pad in front of you, and directly in front of your shoulders. Take hold of the grips with your hands, palms facing up, and slowly squeeze them towards your shoulders before returning to your initial position. Try to keep your chest open and your back in neutral alignment during this exercise.

SEATED TRICEP PUSH-DOWN

Sit facing away from the machine with your feet on the footplate and your hands holding the parallel bars at the side of the machine. You may be provided with an additional footplate that gives you the opportunity to manoeuvre the hand grips into a more comfortable starting position. Keeping your shoulders depressed and your elbows tucked close to your body, slowly push the parallel bars downwards until your arms straighten, then release them upwards again.

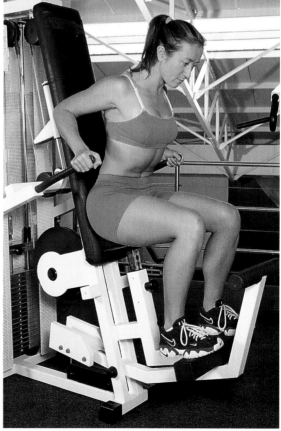

Back

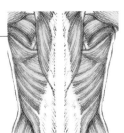

◑ SEATED BACK EXTENSION

Sit with your back against the padded arm and your feet on the footrest. The arm can usually be adjusted to suit your body. Holding onto the seat, slowly push the padded arm backwards as far as you can while remaining comfortable, or until the machine stops you, then return to your starting point. Keep your spine in neutral alignment while performing this exercise.

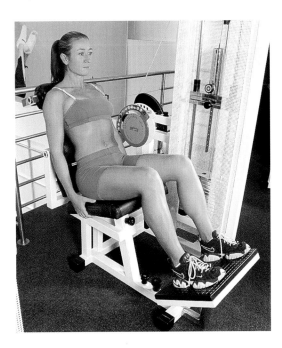

HORIZONTAL HYPEREXTENSION ⮕

Stand with the top of your thighs against the movable pad and your hands holding the grips provided. Slowly lower yourself forwards while hooking your heels under the stationary padded arm, which can be adjusted to suit the length of your legs. With your chest lowered to the floor, release your hands and either clasp in front of or behind your head. Slowly roll your spine upward, one vertebra at a time, until your back is in line with your hips. Roll back down again in the same manner (picture yourself rolling your head towards your pubic bone). Keeping your spine straight in this exercise means you will be bending at the hip instead of in the spine. This works both the back extensor muscles and the buttocks and hamstrings more actively. Although you will also activate the buttocks and hamstrings on the rolling spine action, these will not be the main muscles targeted and so this version is a more significant back exercise. Beginners may prefer to do the seated exercise above.

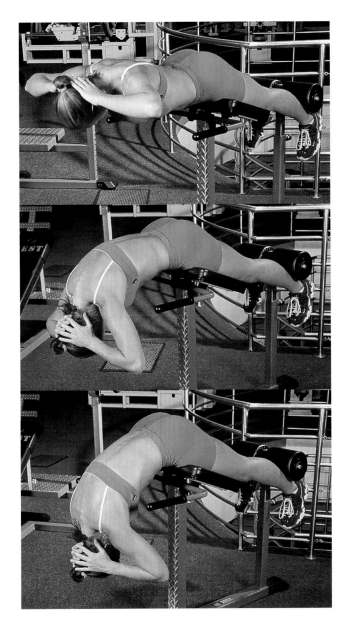

CHIN ASSIST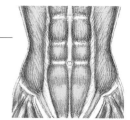

You may need to use quite a few weight plates on this machine if you have never done pull-ups before. Start by using at least half your body weight in plates. The more plates you load on, the easier the exercise becomes. Kneel on the pad provided (sometimes there is a plate intended for standing) facing the machine. Take hold of the grips and pull yourself upward, leading with your chest. Slowly lower to the starting position again. There are usually a number of different grips in different positions from which to choose. Using the wider grip requires more back muscle involvement, while the narrower grip – which you could also do with your palms facing your face – develops the arms more, specifically the biceps.

Abdominals

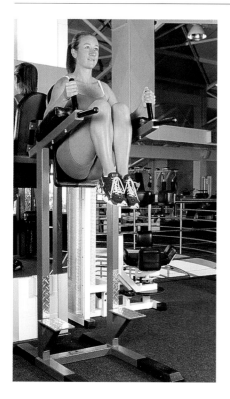

⟲ HANGING KNEE RAISE

With your buttocks leaning against the backrest, your chest upright and your forearms placed onto the arms of the equipment, take hold of the grips and let your feet hang. From here, you can do one of three things:

1. Work the abdominal muscles:
   Raise your knees upward so that they are in line with your hips and use this as your starting point. From here, try to raise the knees as close to the chest as possible before lowering back to your starting point.
2. Work the hip flexors:
   Use the straight-leg hanging position as your starting point, slowly raising your knees to hip height before lowering back to the starting point.
3. Work both the abdominals and the hip flexors by combining the two exercises.

SEATED CRUNCH

Sit in the machine with your feet up on the footrest and the padded arm behind your back (the arm can usually be adjusted to suit your body). Take hold of the handgrips and slowly pull them, and your body, forward toward your knees, before returning to the starting position. Some machines provide a toe grip, creating leverage for pulling the arm forward by means of securing your feet. While you will be able to do more repetitions this way, you would target the abdominals far more actively without hooking your toes, which prevents your hip flexors from assisting significantly.

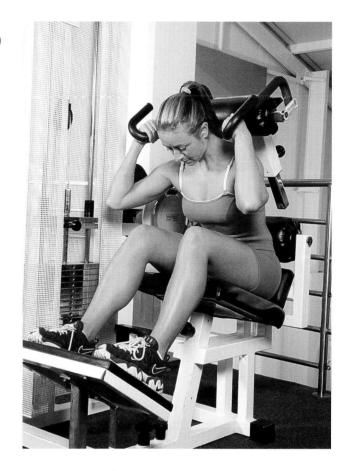

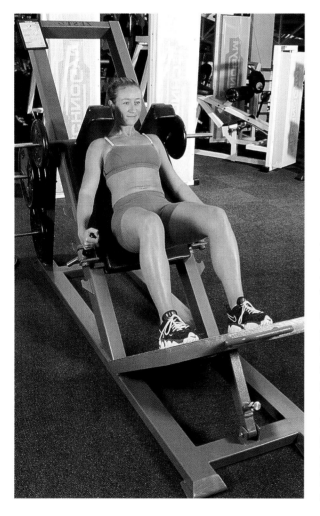

Legs and buttocks

HACK SQUATS

Stand facing away from the machine, with your feet placed towards the front of the adjustable footplate, approximately shoulder-width apart. Your back should be resting against the padded area and your shoulders under the horizontal padded arms. Push against the shoulder pads so that you are holding the load with your legs, then release the brake at the side of the machine. Slowly bend your knees, lowering your body into a squat (see page 85) before returning to your initial position. Try not to work too heavy with too deep a knee bend in this exercise, as knee pain can develop with excessive strain on the joint. Remember to replace the brake before attempting to climb out of this machine.

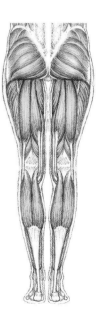

LYING LEG PRESS

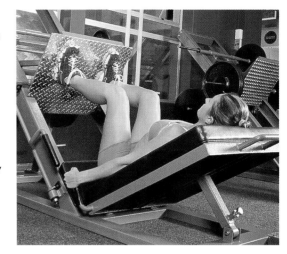

Sit facing the machine with your knees bent and feet placed towards the front of the footplate, approximately shoulder-width apart. Your back and head should be resting against the adjustable padded plate. Push against the footplate, so that you are holding the load with your legs, before releasing the brake at the side of the machine. Then slowly straighten your legs before lowering back to a point where your knees are close to your chest. As with the hack squats, try not to work too heavy with too deep a knee bend, and remember to replace the brake before attempting to climb out of the machine.

LEG EXTENSION

Sit in the padded seat with your shins tucked under the padded arm, which can usually be adjusted to suit the length of your legs, and your hands holding the grips at the side of the machine. Your back should be resting against the backrest unless the seat is too long and you find you are slouching; in this case rather sit up straight, away from the backrest. Slowly raise the padded arm until your knees are straight, then lower back to the starting position. Be sure to keep your spine in neutral alignment, as it has a tendency to round in the lower back when the quadriceps are activated.

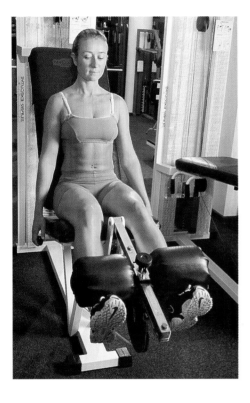

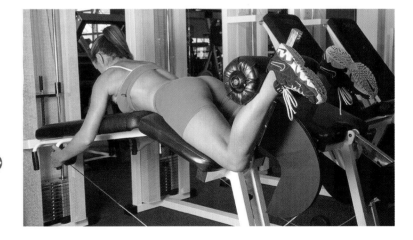

LYING HAM CURL

Lie face down on the machine with your heels tucked under the padded arm, which can usually be adjusted to suit the length of your legs, and your hands holding the grips at the side of the machine. Slowly lift your heels toward your buttocks, ensuring that both your chest and pelvis remain firmly against the bench. (The pelvis, in particular, has a tendency to lift off when the hamstrings are activated.) Flexing your feet during this exercise will isolate the hamstrings further, since you will be eliminating calf assistance. Lower back to the starting point again.

INNER THIGH (ADDUCTOR) ➜

Sit in the padded seat with your inner knees placed against the padded knee-rests (which will be wide), your feet on the footplates and your hands holding the grips at the side of the machine. At the same time, rest your back against the backrest and keep your head straight. To begin the exercise, slowly bring your legs toward one another as much as possible before releasing back out to the starting position. Be sure that you keep neutral alignment of your spine throughout this exercise. Take your legs only as wide as feels comfortable for you. If the machine takes them too wide and you struggle to close them from the fully open position, either reduce the number of weights you are using, or only open them halfway until your strength increases.

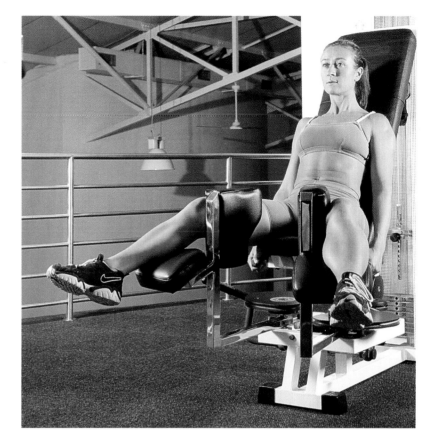

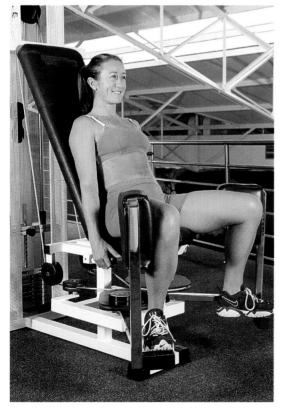

⬅ OUTER THIGH (ABDUCTOR)

This exercise is the exact reverse of the inner thigh (adductor) exercise described above. Sit in the padded seat with your outer knees placed against the padded knee-rests, your feet on the footplates and your hands holding the grips at the side of the machine. Rest your back against the backrest. Slowly take your legs out sideways as far apart as possible before bringing them back to the starting position once more. Again, as in the previous exercise, be sure that you maintain neutral alignment of your spine throughout this exercise.

You may find that you do not initially have the strength to take your legs as wide as the machine will allow. Keep your resistance/weight low and use the full range of the machine, rather than working with too heavy a load and only using a small range of motion.

Further Reading

Anon. (2001). *Energise Your Life*. London: Duncain Baird Publishers.

Anon. (2003). *Synergize: The Dynamic Mind and Body Workout*. London: Hamlyn.

Belling, N. (2003). *The Yoga Handbook*. Cape Town: New Holland Publishers.

Briffa, J. (2002). *Ultimate Health*. London: Penguin Group.

Cochram, S. and House, T. (2000). *Stronger Arms and Upper Body*. USA: Human Kinetics.

Dalgleish, J. and Dollery, S. (2001). *The Health & Fitness Handbook*. Essex: Pearson Education Limited.

Graham, H. (2002). *The Lazy Man's Guide to Exercise*. Dublin: New Leaf.

Green, B. (2002). *Get with the Program*. New York: Simon & Schuster.

Holford, P. (1997). *Optimum Nutrition Bible*. London: Piatkus.

Holford, P. (1998). *100% Health*. London: Piatkus.

Malcolm, L. (2001). *Health Style*. London: Duncain Baird Publishers.

Menezes, A. (1998). *Complete Guide to Joseph H. Pilates Techniques of Physical Conditioning*. Australia: Hunter House.

Ungaro, A. (2002). *Pilates Body in Motion*. London: Dorling Kindersley.

Urla, J. (2002). *Yogilates*. London: Thorsons.

Websites

www.fitnesszone.co.za
An excellent site. Loads of information covering all aspects of health, fitness and nutrition. Allows you to pose questions to a fitness expert. Books and videos are also on offer.

www.acefitness.org
Another good site covering all aspects of health, nutrition and fitness. Although it deals more with the education of fitness practitioners, it also provides vast amounts of information for the layman.

www.anatomical.com
Charts relating to anatomy, training heart rates, weight training illustrations, alternative health therapies, health education, etc. Videos and books also available.

www.ciavideo.com
Videos of workouts by various presenters in the United States – great for exercising at home.

www.musclemedia.com
Specifics regarding weight-training issues. Back orders of magazines are also available, as well as information on nutrition for weight training.

www.sportsci.org
Although this is a very scientific site, there are some good articles on research relating to various sports and the issues affecting them, such as hydration, training, nutrition, etc.

www.turnstep.com
Good for ordering exercise videos. Some articles of interest are included, but are more for instructors.

www.ideafit.com
Although mainly aimed at fitness instructors and trainers, this site includes articles the layperson may find interesting and valuable – go to 'publications'.

www.topendsports.com/testing/
This site relates specifically to fitness testing. Tests range from very scientific to home-based and easy to use. Also lists various fitness-related books.

http://primusweb.com/fitnesspartner/index.html
Lists various fitness-related sites and relevant articles.

www.dolfzine.com
Huge range of articles covering issues such as training, nutrition, dieting, exercise and pregnancy, yoga, Pilates, how to choose a personal trainer, and so on.

http://groups.yahoo.com/group/Supertraining/
This site is devoted to sports, strength and fitness science, as well as training, therapy and education. You will need to join the group in order to access the information posted.

www.fitpro.com
Primarily aimed at fitness practitioners, but also has some good articles for the layperson, covering a wide range of health and fitness-related topics.

Glossary

Anterior pelvic tilt: bottom of the pelvis (pubic bone) tilts back while the top of the pelvis (hip bones) tilts forward

Ballistic: to bounce or jerk (in the context of flexibility training)

Body mass index (BMI): calculation of the body's total mass, using weight and height values

Cardiovascular endurance: body's ability to perform continuous exercise at an elevated heart rate for long periods

Compound exercises: exercises that significantly target more than one muscle at a time

Continuous training: cardiovascular activity that is constant in effort

Contraction: the action of shortening a muscle

Cross training: combining various exercise types and intensities

Ectomorph: long, lean body type

Endomorph: high fat-storing, heavier body type

External rotation: outward rotation of a limb

Fartlek training: non-measured or random periods of high- and low-intensity exercise

Fast twitch: type of muscle fibre that contracts quickly, so is suited to short, sharp bursts of exercise

Flexibility training: a method of training that serves to increase the range of movement around a joint

Frequency: number of times an activity is repeated

Functional abdominal training: training abdominals in a manner that mimics everyday movements more closely

Glycaemix index: indicator of how slowly or quickly the glucose in carbohydrate foods is released into the bloodstream

High impact: type of activity that may have both of the feet off the ground at any given time

High intensity: activity that requires high levels of effort, resulting in higher heart rates

Internal rotation: inward rotation of a limb

Interval training: repetitive, measured cycles of rest and effort

Isolation exercises: exercises that significantly target one muscle at a time

Kyphosis: abnormal curvature of spine, resulting in hunched back appearance

Low impact: type of activity that always has one foot in contact with the ground

Low intensity: activity that requires low levels of effort, resulting in lower heart rates

Maximum heart rate: the highest number of times your heart can beat in a minute

Mesomorph: muscular, athletic body type

Momentum: uncontrolled, often swinging movement by the body or limbs

Muscle imbalance: unequal strength in a muscle or muscle group, resulting in one muscle or muscle group being stronger or weaker than another

Muscular endurance: ability of muscles to perform many contractions against a load without fatiguing; can also be used to describe the amount of time a contraction can be held without fatiguing

Muscular strength: maximum amount of force a muscle or group of muscles can produce in a single contraction

Neutral pelvis: pelvis tilted neither forward, nor backward; an optimal position

Non-weight-bearing exercise: activities that suspend the body, so it does not act against gravity

Overload: challenging body with a higher load than it is used to

Perceived scale of exertion: personal awareness of effort levels

Posterior pelvic tilt: bottom of pelvis (pubic bone) tilts forward, while the top of the pelvis (hip bones) tilts backward

Repetitions: in the context of resistance training, the number of times you repeat a specific muscle contraction or complete a specific exercise

Resistance training: working against load or resistance – either an external load or your own body weight

Resting heart rate: measurement of the number of times the heart beats per minute when at rest

Reversibility: the principle stating that unless you consistently challenge the body, it will lose its adaptation response to training

Set: a group of repetitions

Slow twitch: type of muscle fibre that contracts slowly so is suited to endurance activities

Specificity: principle of matching specific training exercises to specific goals or activities

Split routine: exercising some parts of the body on one day and other parts on another day

Standard routine: exercising the whole body on one day

Torso: trunk, including chest, abdomen and back

Torso stabilization: developing strength in the torso muscles

Weight training: working against an external load or resistance

Weight-bearing exercise: any type of activity that causes the body to act against gravity

Index

Bold numbers refer to pictures and main entries.